LEFT VENTRICULAR HYPERTROPHY

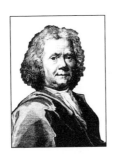

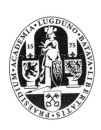

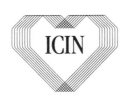

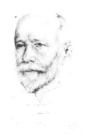

WILLEM EINTHOVEN
1860-1927

Developments in Cardiovascular Medicine

VOLUME 223

Left Ventricular Hypertrophy

Physiology versus Pathology

by

ERNST E. VAN DER WALL

ARNOUD VAN DER LAARSE

BABETTE M. PLUIM

and

ALBERT V.G. BRUSCHKE
Leiden University Medical Center,
Leiden, The Netherlands

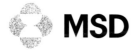

KLUWER ACADEMIC PUBLISHERS
DORDRECHT / BOSTON / LONDON

A C.I.P. Catalogue record for this book is available from the Library of Congress

ISBN 0-7923-6038-9

Published by Kluwer Academic Publishers,
P.O. Box 17, 3300 AA Dordrecht, The Netherlands.

Sold and distributed in North, Central and South America
by Kluwer Academic Publishers,
101 Philip Drive, Norwell, MA 02061, U.S.A.

In all other countries, sold and distributed
by Kluwer Academic Publishers,
P.O. Box 322, 3300 AH Dordrecht, The Netherlands.

Printed on acid-free paper

TABLE OF CONTENTS

FOREWORD

The importance of left ventricular hypertrophy in cardiovascular disease has gained wide recognition. Left ventricular hypertrophy is a highly important risk factor associated with major cardiovascular events, including symptomatic heart failure, particularly in patients with systemic hypertension. Over the past years much has been learned about the genetics, molecular background, prevalence, incidence and prognosis of left ventricular hypertrophy. A variety of noninvasive methods has emerged for detecting left ventricular hypertrophy and the assessment of reversal of hypertrophy. Yet, a lot of controversy remains about the connotations and clinical implications of left ventricular hypertrophy. For instance, in the athlete's heart left ventricular hypertrophy may constitute a physiological adaptation to pressure overload, which normalizes following discontinuation of strenuous physical activity. On the other hand, in particular in patients with hypertension, left ventricular hypertrophy denotes a serious prognosis in the course of hypertension. In these patients left ventricular hypertrophy should be regarded as a grave prognostic sign rather than an innocent compensatory phenomenon. The distinction between physiologic and pathophysiologic left ventricular hypertrophy has been the basis for this book.

Basically, the interest for left ventricular hypertrophy in our institution (Leiden University Medical Center) dates back to 1992 when we received a large investment grant from NWO (Nederlands Wetenschappelijk Onderzoek, Dutch Scientific Investigation) to perform magnetic resonance imaging and spectoscopy to evaluate individuals with left ventricular hypertrophy. At that time, we decided to focus on three different groups of individuals with left ventricular hypertrophy: elite athletes, patients with hypertension, and patients with aortic valve disease. In this way approached, we tried to get an answer on the issue whether one could distinguish between physiologic and pathologic left ventricular hypertrophy. This was a large project involving both the Departments of Cardiology and Radiology of our institution, and the full-time involvement of three research fellows. The project was also supported by the Ministry of Welfare, Health and Culture (WVC), the Netherlands Heart Foundation (NHS), and the Interuniversity Cardiology Institute of The Netherlands (ICIN), the latter being an institute of the Royal Netherlands Academy of Arts and Sciences. The project, as described in the grant, was almost completed in 1998 and at that time it was decided that we would organize a special meeting around the topic left ventricular hypertrophy.

Left ventricular hypertrophy - physiology versus pathology is a bibliographical reflection of a Boerhaave Symposium held on April 9, 1999, Leiden, The Netherlands. At this symposium the major issues dealing with left ventricular hypertrophy were discussed from etiology, genetics, detection, and therapy of left ventricular hypertrophy. In particular, the book includes novel detection methods for left ventricular hypertrophy such as magnetic resonance imaging and spectroscopy. Furthermore, much attention was paid to the molecular and genetic approach of left ventricular hypertrophy. In the last chapter the clinical relevance of genotype in the context of hypertrophy is described. This chapter was composed by Prof.dr. K. Schwartz, who gave the illustrious Einthoven Lecture 1999 at the end of the symposium. The Einthoven Lecture is named after Willem Einthoven, who was awarded the Nobel Prize in 1924 for inventing the electrocardiogram. Every two years the prestigious Einthoven Lecture is presented at our university by a well-known national or international expert in the field of cardiovascular diseases.

The publication of the book would not have been possible without a generous educational grant from Merck, Sharp and Dohme (Haarlem, The Netherlands). We like to acknowledge the efforts of the authors, all of whom have written dedicated and well-focused chapters. We also like to thank the Boerhaave Committee (Mrs. L. Zitter) who put a lot of effort in preparation of the manuscript, and gave permission to publish this book. Lastly, we are grateful for the support by Mrs. Amber Tanghe-Neely (Kluwer Academic Publishers, Dordrecht) for proper guiding of the book preparation, and Mr. Jan Schoones (Leiden Medical Library) who checked all the chapter references and took care of the Index.

We hope that our book will assist the clinical cardiologist, the fellows in cardiology, the general internist, the radiologist, the cardiothoracic surgeon, the biochemist, the physiologist, the pharmacologist, and the basic research fellow, in understanding the most recent insights in the background of physiologic versus pathologic left ventricular hypertrophy.

The Editors

Ernst E. van der Wall
Arnoud van der Laarse
Babette M. Pluim
Albert V.G. Bruschke

LIST OF CONTRIBUTORS

L.H.B. Baur
Department of Cardiology, Leiden University Medical Center
Albinusdreef 2, P.O. Box 9600, 2300 RC Leiden, The Netherlands
Co-authors: A.V.G. Bruschke, J. Braun, M. Hazekamp, Y. Houdas, H.A.Huysmans X.Y. Jin, A.P. Kappetein, C.H. Peels, E.A. van der Velde, E.E. van der Wall

A.J. Brees
Department of Cardiology, Leiden University Medical Center
Albinusdreef 2, P.O. Box 9600, 2300 RC Leiden, The Netherlands
Co-authors: B.M.Pluim, H. Lamb, A. de Roos, H.W. Vliegen, E.E. van der Wall

P.A.F.M. Doevendans
Department of Cardiology, Academic Hospital Maastricht
P. Debyelaan 25, 6202 AZ Maastricht, The Netherlands
Co-authors: R. Bronsaer, J.M. van Dantzig

D.G.J.M. Duncker
Department of Experimental Cardiology, Erasmus University Rotterdam
P.O. Box 1738, 3000 DR Rotterdam, The Netherlands

A. van der Laarse
Department of Cardiology, Leiden University Medical Center
Albinusdreef 2, P.O. Box 9600, 2300 RC Leiden, The Netherlands
Co-authors: A.V.G. Bruschke, C. Ruwhof, E.E. van der Wall, J.E.T. van Wamel

H. J. Lamb
Department of Radiology, Leiden University Medical Center
Albinusdreef 2, P.O. Box 9600, 2300 RC Leiden, The Netherlands
Co-authors: A. de Roos, E.E. van der Wall

B.M. Pluim

Royal Netherlands Lawn Tennis Association, Sports Medical Center Papendal, Papendallaan 60, 6816 VD Arnhem, The Netherlands

Co-authors: A.V.G. Bruschke, A. van der Laarse, H.W. Vliegen, E.E. van der Wall

J.J. Schipperheijn

Department of Cardiology, Leiden University Medical Center

Albinusdreef 2, P.O. Box 9600, 2300 RC Leiden, The Netherlands

K. Schwartz, Directeur de Recherce INSERM/CNRS

INSERM, U 153, 47, Boulevard de l'Hôpital, 75651 Paris Cedex 13, France

R.A. Tio

Department of Clinical Pharmacology, University Groningen

Ant. Deusinglaan 1, 9713 AV Groningen, The Netherlands

Co-authors: R. de Boer, W.H. van Gilst, D.J. van Veldhuisen

A.A.M. Wilde

Department of Cardiology, Amsterdam Medical Center

Meibergdreef 9, 1105 AZ Amsterdam, The Netherlands

1.   ETIOLOGY OF LEFT VENTRICULAR HYPERTROPHY

A. VAN DER LAARSE, C. RUWHOF, J.E.T. VAN WAMEL, E.E. VAN
DER WALL, A.V.G. BRUSCHKE

Summary

In the etiology of left ventricular hypertrophy, left ventricular overload is "transduced" to the myocardial tissue by physical forces, such as stretch, imposed to myocardial cells, followed by biological effects mediated through one or more mechano-chemical coupling systems. Several candidate components of such systems are 1)membrane proteins, such as stretch-activated cation channels, 2) growth factors that are released from cells upon stretch, and 3) integrin receptor activation. The hypertrophic phenotypes, being highly dependent upon the stimulus that caused hypertrophy, may express "fetal" genes and downregulation of constitutively expressed genes. Besides cardiomyocytes, other cell types in the myocardium are sensitive to overload. Fibroblasts proliferate and are responsible for compositional and structural changes in the extracellular matrix, probably stimulated to do so by increased neurohumoral activation. During the development of myocardial hypertrophy, angiogenesis and vasculogenesis should accompany the growth of myocytes. Vascular cell types, such as endothelial cells and smooth muscle cells, are sensitive to mechanical forces like mechanical activity, stretch, and shear stress. However, the appropriate growth of arteries, arterioles and capillaries may be hampered by insufficient angiogenesis, thickening of the vessel wall, and collagen accumulation in the arterioles. These overload-induced alterations of left ventricular cells and matrix may lead to diastolic and systolic dysfunction and arrhythmogenesis.

Introduction

In the postnatal mammalian heart cardiac overload as well as increased mechanical activity of the heart induces a growth response in myocytes, being limited to cellular hypertrophy as

E. E. van der Wall et al.(eds.), Left Ventricular Hypertrophy, 1-13.
© 1999 *Kluwer Academic Publishers. Printed in the Netherlands.*

these cells have lost their ability to divide. To maintain proper myocardial structure and blood supply, matrix protein synthesizing cells, such as fibroblasts, divide and vasculogenesis takes place. The result is a heart with increased weight due to an increase in mass of one or more cardiac compartments. Although it is tempting to compare a hypertrophic heart of a 70 kg person to a normal heart of a 90 kg person, such a comparison should be restricted to hearts with "physiological" hypertrophy, as present in athletes and cyclists (see Chapter 7 by Pluim et al. on the athlete's heart). Whether due to intermittent (as in athletes) or continuous cardiac overloading (as in hypertensives), patients with cardiac pressure or volume overload have hypertrophic hearts with characteristics that widely differ from those of normal hearts. During the past two decades, particularly molecular-biological investigations have shed light on the alterations in cellular phenotypes of myocytes of overloaded hearts, including human hearts. These phenotypes are dependent on the stimulus that caused hypertrophy and may be the result of a genetically limited range of responses available to adult cardiac myocytes in the process of adapting to changes in mechanical load or activity.

Origin of the hypertrophic response

Pressure overload and volume overload cause different myocardial phenotypes. Stimulation of quiescent isolated adult myocytes causes a hypertrophic phenotype. Apart from these load-dependent and mechanical activity-dependent myocardial hypertrophy models, a number of hormones (α_1-adrenoceptor agonists, growth hormone), vasoactive substances (endothelin-1, prostaglandin $F_{2\alpha}$, angiotensinII), growth factors (bFGF, PDGF, TGF$_\beta$, IGF-I, IGF-II) and cytokines (IL-1, IL-6, cardiotrophin-1) induce myocardial hypertrophy. Therefore, it is likely that physical factors associated with load and mechanical activity share signal transduction pathways with the substances mentioned earlier. However, in comparison with the vast knowledge about receptor stimulation and cellular signal transduction, little is known about the ways physical factors are relayed to the interior of the cell. A mechano-chemical coupling system must exist that induces biological effects, such as hypertrophy and proliferation. Candidates for such a coupling system are 1) membrane proteins, such as ion channels, ion exchangers and membrane-associated enzymes, that become activated if the membrane is stretched or deformed, 2) stretch-induced release of growth factors, hormones and cytokines, and 3) integrin receptor activation.

Mechano-sensitive membrane proteins

Stretch-activated ion channels, such as cation channels, are present in mammalian cardiomyocytes.[1] The open probability (P_o) for Ca^{2+} ions increases upon stretch. Distortion of the sarcolemma by pushing a blunt microelectrode onto the myocyte's surface causes a rapid increase of intracellular Ca^{2+} concentration ($[Ca^{2+}]_i$).[2] However, a specific inhibitor of the stretch-activated cation channels, gadolinium, was unable to inhibit stretch-induced oncogene expression and protein synthesis.[3,4] Although the latter results appear to disqualify the stretch-activated cation channels as the primary mechano-chemical coupler, recent findings by Molkentin and coworkers demonstrate that an increased $[Ca^{2+}]_i$ is an important mediator of angiotensin-II and endothelin-1 induced cardiac hypertrophy by activating a calcium/calmodulin-dependent phosphatase, calcineurin.[5] Calcineurin dephosphorylates the transcription factor NF-AT3, enabling to translocate to the nucleus where cardiac transcription is activated. Also Shadoshima and Izumo provided evidence that an increased $[Ca^{2+}]_i$ is a codeterminant of stretch-induced hypertrophy.[6] They demonstrated that buffering intracellular Ca^{2+} ions by membrane-permeable BAPTA-AM attenuated stretch-induced oncogen expression.

Another mechanosensitive membrane protein is the Na^+/H^+-exchanger, that may be related to integrin receptor activation (see later). Activation of the Na^+/H^+-exchanger will increase H^+ efflux and Na^+ influx, which may result in an increase of Ca^{2+} influx by the Na^+/Ca^{2+}-exchanger. A specific inhibitor of the Na^+/H^+-exchanger, HOE694, drastically inhibited stretch-induced hypertrophic responses, including signalling and protein synthesis.[4] Whether the Na^+/H^+-exchanger-induced alkalinization, increase of $[Na^+]_i$ or secondary increase of $[Ca^{2+}]_i$ is responsible for facilitation of hypertrophy to occur is not completely clear, but in view of the results mentioned in the previous paragraph we wish to stress the importance of an increased $[Ca^{2+}]_i$ as a codeterminant.

Other membrane proteins that may respond to stretch are phospholipases. Myocardial overload or myocyte stretch are associated with increased activity of phospholipase C.[6,7] The stretch-induced increases of cellular IP_3 concentration (within 1-2 minutes) and of c-*fos* expression (after 30 minutes) were completely suppressed by D609, an inhibitor of phospholipase C. The phospholipase C-catalyzed reaction leads to formation of IP_3 and diacylglycerol. The latter, reaching a maximal level after 5 minutes of stretch, activates protein kinase C (PKC). PKC activity was doubled by stretch, and its activation persisted for at least 30 minutes.[6] The stretch-induced c-*fos* expression was completely suppressed by inhibitors of PKC, such as H-7 and staurosporin, as well as by inactivation of PKC due to 24 hours pretreatment with phorbolester.[6] PKC is an important representative of cellular signalling proteins, and is also activated by all phospholipase C-coupled receptors for endogenous mediators of hypertrophic growth, such as angiotensin-II, endothelin-1 and α_1-adrenoceptor agonists.

Stretch-induced release of growth factors, hormones and cytokines

Several receptor agonists (growth factors, hormones and cytokines) are produced by myocardial cells (myocytes, fibroblasts, vascular smooth muscle cells, vascular endothelial cells) themselves and are released upon overload or stretch. Upon release, these factors may stimulate the same cell or other cells (autocrine and paracrine effects, respectively) resulting in amplification of hypertrophic stimuli. The release of peptides from stretched myocytes has been shown to occur through transient membrane disruptions caused by membrane stretch.[8,9]

Fibroblast growth factor. The isolated Langendorff-perfused rat heart releases acidic fibroblast growth factor (aFGF) and basic FGF (bFGF) and this release is stimulated by positive inotropic interventions[9] or by pacing of quiescent adult myocytes.[8] The hypertrophic phenotype induced by bFGF is quite similar to that induced by pressure overload[10] and includes increased expression of smooth muscle (SM) α-actin and skeletal (SK) α-actin.[11,12]

Transforming growth factor-ß. Myocardial TGFß expression is increased in several experimental models of pressure and volume overload.[13-15] The myocardial fibroblasts are considered responsible for most of the TGFß production.[16] The paracrine effects of TGFß are: myocyte hypertrophy with reintroduction of the fetal program of gene transcription, including induction of SK α-actin, ß-myosin heavy chain (ßMHC) and atrial natriuretic peptide (ANP).[17,18]

Endothelin-1. ET-1, a peptide originally found in endothelial cells, is a strong stimulus for myocyte hypertrophy[19,20] with enhanced expression of muscle-specific genes, such as myosin light chain-1 (MLC2), SK α-actin and SK troponin-I.[21] In the rat after aortic constriction, plasma ET-1 levels increased, peaked at 24 hours, and returned to basal levels at 4 days.[22] PreproET-1 mRNA levels in left ventricular myocardium are increased 24 hours after aortic constriction, and declined to basal levels at 4 days. Suzuki et al.[23] and Harada et al.[24] demonstrated that ET-1 produced by fibroblasts stimulated myocyte hypertrophy. An ET$_A$-receptor antagonist, BQ123, blocked the hypertrophic responses of myocytes exposed to conditioned medium of nonmuscle cells. These results demonstrate that nonmuscle cells in myocardial tissue regulate myocyte hypertrophy, at least partly via ET-1 secretion. If BQ123 was adminstered by minipump to rats, starting 24 hours before aortic constriction, the aortic constriction-induced increase in left ventricular weight and myocyte size was blocked in the first week, but not after 2 weeks.[22] So, the inhibitory effect of BQ123 is restricted to the first week, and it may be speculated that cardiac ET-1 may act as an "initiating" hypertrophy factor during the early phase of pressure overload. However, other factors, such as local renin-angiotensin systems and several growth factors may take over as a "maintaining" factor during the late phase of pressure overload.

Angiotensin-II. Angiotensin-II is produced by cardiomyocytes and is released upon stretch.[25] No secretion of angiotensin-II from fibroblasts was observed. Stretch upregulated myocyte angiotensinogen gene expression by a factor of 4.8 in 24 hours.[25,26] The dissociation of the effects of angiotensin-II on hypertension and hypertrophy has been demonstrated by Linz et al.[27,28] They showed that in hypertensive rats high doses of ramipril (1 mg/kg) regressed both hypertension and hypertrophy, whereas low doses of ramipril (10 µg/kg) had no effect on hypertension but regressed hypertrophy. The results of Sadoshima et al.[25] were not corroborated by those of other groups, which showed that angiotensin-II-induced myocardial hypertrophy is mediated by fibroblasts, having considerably more AT$_1$-receptors than myocytes.[29-31]

Integrin receptor stimulation

The primary receptors that link cells to the extracellular matrix (ECM) are integrins. Via these receptors cell shape is controlled, and cell shape in turn controls survival and growth.[32] Mechanical stretch is, probably by mechanochemical coupling, transduced to the interior of the cell by stimulation of integrin receptors which connect the ECM to the cytoskeletal network. Upon binding of an integrin ligand to the integrin receptor, the integrin-receptor complex binds to various proteins of the ECM, while a short cytoplasmic domain has been shown to interact with the cytoskeleton in the cell. Integrins can transmit signals not only by organizing the cytoskeleton, but also by altering biochemical properties such as the extent of tyrosine phosphorylation of a complex of proteins including pp125[FAK] (FAK stands for focal adhesion kinase). Since cytoskeletal proteins can potentially regulate plasma membrane proteins such as enzymes, ion channels and ion exchangers, mechanical stress could modulate these membrane-associated proteins and stimulate second messenger systems through the cytoskeleton. Wang et al. showed that integrin β_1 not only induced focal adhesion formation, but also supported a force-dependent stiffening response and that an increase in the cytoskeletal stiffness to the applied stress required the intact cytoskeleton.[33] Their results suggest that mechanical stress is first received by integrins, and that next interlinked actin myofilaments transduces mechanical stress in concert with microtubules and intermediate filaments. Tsutsui et al.[34] have provided evidence that pressure loading increases the microtubule compartment (by polymerized tubulin) of the cardiac muscle cell cytoskeleton which was responsible for the cellular contractile dysfunction observed. They suggested that the microtubule component of the cytoskeleton imposes a resistive intracellular load of the shortening sarcomere rather than altering the stiffness of the sarcomere-sarcolemma connections. An excess of microtubules in stress-hypertrophied cells increases this load and impedes sarcomere motion. If the technique of differential RNA display was used to compare mRNA transcripts from control hearts and hearts of guinea-pigs with aortic constriction, mRNA of titin (a sarcomeric cytoskeletal protein), desmin and tubulin were increased during development of compensated left ventricular pressure overload hypertrophy. After transition to decompensated congestive heart failure, titin mRNA declined, but desmin and tubulin mRNA remained elevated.[35] Besides an increased synthesis of microtubular proteins, the increased microtubule density appears to be due to microtubule stabilization, caused by sequential, time-dependent posttranslational modifications of tubulin.[36]

The "hypertrophic" cellular phenotypes

Within 30 minutes of exposure of myocytes to a hypertrophic stimulus early response genes, such as c-*fos*, c-*jun* and c-*myc*, are activated. After 6-12 hours, genes that normally are expressed in fetal hearts only are induced, such as ß-MHC (in rodents), SK α-actin, ß-tropomyosin, ANP and the α_3-subunit of Na$^+$,K$^+$-ATPase. After 12-24 hours constitutively expressed genes become upregulated, including those encoding MLC-2 and cardiac α-actin. After 24 hours the increased rate of protein synthesis starts to increase myocyte dimensions. The sets of reintroduced genes and upregulated constitutively expressed genes are dependent of the stimulus that caused hypertrophy. Also the morphology of the myocytes may differ among the models of hypertrophy research. Synthesis of sarcomeres in series with existing sarcomeres leads to increased myocyte width as is observed in pressure overloaded myocardium, whereas synthesis of sarcomeres parallel to existing sarcomeres leads to increased myocyte length as is observed in volume overloaded myocardium. As to functional consequences of alterations in myocyte phenotype, several "adaptations" regarding proteins involved in calcium handling (for instance, sarcoplasmic reticulum Ca^{2+}-ATPase, or SERCA2), and proteins involved in transmembrane ion movements (for instance ion channels and ion exchangers) may lead to systolic dysfunction[37] and arrhythmogenesis.[38]

Besides myocytes, other myocardial cells, the so-called nonmuscle cells, respond to increased load and mechanical activity. Fibroblasts, vascular smooth muscle cells and vascular endothelial cells are also sensitive to increased load and stretch. Fibroblasts proliferate in response to these conditions, thereby maintaining normal cell density per gram of myocardium. In a study by Vliegen et al.[39] on 43 *post-mortem* human hearts, the number of connective tissue cells per heart correlated well to indexed heart weight (r=0.76, p<0.001), but the number of connective tissue cells per gram of heart weight was hardly dependent upon the extent of hypertrophy. Myocardial fibroblasts are extremely sensitive to stretch. Stretch-induced effects are induction of oncogenes (c-*fos*, c-*jun*, *fra*-1) within 1 hour, and increased rate of protein synthesis in the first 2 hours.[40] The role of fibroblasts in producing substances with paracrine effects on myocytes has been mentioned above, and we have corroborated these findings by demonstrating that myocytes exposed to conditioned medium of stretched fibroblasts had increased oncogene (c-*fos*, c-*jun*, *fra*-1) expression within 1 hour, increased ANP expression within 1 hour, and increased rate of protein synthesis in the first 4 hours.[40] Recently, McKenna[41] et al. showed that cardiac fibroblasts respond to stretch by cellular signalling in a way that is dependent upon matrix composition and integrin receptors. Integrin-matrix interactions were considered to be the mechanotransducer of stretch that transforms mechanical stimuli into chemical signals.

Growth of vascular cells

In the vascular wall pulsatile stretch stimulates proliferation of vascular smooth muscle cells.[42,43] Hishikawa et al. demonstrated that pulsatile stretch of human coronary artery smooth muscle cells in culture caused superoxide anion production that could be blocked by NADPH oxidase inhibitors.[44] The consequences of increased oxidative stress were a sustained activation of nuclear factor-κB (NF-κB) for up to 24 hours, an increase in DNA synthesis, and cell proliferation. The sustained activation of NF-κB, increased DNA synthesis and cell proliferation were abolished by cotreatment with antioxidants, such as N-acetylcysteine.

The effects of stretch on vascular endothelial cells have been studied extensively. Pulsatile stretch induced endothelial cell proliferation,[45] associated with increased tissue-plasminogen activator (tPA) mRNA as well as tPA release,[46] increased ecNOS mRNA and ecNOS protein levels,[47,48] increased expression of monocyte chemotactic protein-1,[49] increased expression of PDGF-B chain,[50] increased expression of ICAM-1 mRNA,[51] and increased ET-1 mRNA and ET-1 secretion, both being dependent upon protein kinase C and intracellular Ca^{2+} ions.[52,53] Using whole heart stretch by inflating a balloon in the left ventricle of an isolated perfused rat heart for 30 minutes, VEGF mRNA was upregulated considerably in the stretched left ventricle as well as in the unstretched right ventricle.[54] This stretch-induced VEGF expression was blocked by an anti-TGFß antibody, but not by ET_A- and AT_1-receptor antagonists. Perfusing the heart with coronary venous effluent collected from the stretched heart was able to induce VEGF expression, as was true for hearts perfused with buffer to which TGFß was added. The finding that the stretch-induced increase of VEGF expression in the heart is mediated, at least in part, by TGFß, emphasizes the role of paracrine factors in potentiating, modulating or sustaining the signals initiated in the myocardium by load itself. We have demonstrated that conditioned medium of endothelial cells stretched for 15-60 minutes caused an increase in oncogen expression and ANP expression in stationary myocytes (unpublished observations).

It seems unlikely that during development of cardiac hypertrophy vasculogenesis and angiogenesis are started and maintained by stretch only. Besides vascular stretch, an increase in fluid shear stress may be responsible for upregulation of adhesion molecules (e.g. ICAM-1) and chemotactic factors (e.g. MCP-1) that cause monocytes to invade the vascular wall and, by producing growth factors, promote vasculogenesis and angiogenesis. For vasculogenesis to occur, the vessel wall should undergo "controlled destruction" to create space for new cells.[55] Activation of matrix metalloproteinases, necrosis and apoptosis are components of the destruction process that is followed by proliferation of smooth muscle cells to build a normal wall thickness-to-diameter ratio of the mature but larger vessel.

In **pressure-overloaded** myocardium of experimental animals and of humans, capillary growth was inadequate leading to a decrease of capillary density and capillary/fiber ratio.[56,57] The increase in minimal coronary resistance was mainly due to thickening of arteriolar walls and restriction of their maximal dilatation by increased collagen accumulation.[58,59] In **volume-overloaded** myocardium, capillary growth appears to be adequate as is arteriolar density.[60] The role of mechanical factors in capillary growth has been reviewed by Hudlicka and Brown and the factors implicated are increased mechanical activity, stretch and shear stress.[61]

Growth of the interstitial compartment

The cardiac interstitium contains connective tissue cells and a structural protein network, called the extracellular matrix (ECM), mainly consisting of collagen types I and III, and elastin. The function of the ECM is to support and align the cellular structures (myocytes, capillaries, lymph vessels) relative to one another, thereby preserving myocardial architecture. By preventing muscle fiber and cardiomyocyte slippage, myocyte-generated force is transduced to the ventricular chamber. ECM also protects the myocytes from overstretch.

In ventricular hypertrophy caused by **volume-overload** or by thyroxine administration, myocardial collagen concentration remains unchanged. In left ventricular **pressure-overload** hypertrophy, however, an increase in myocardial collagen concentration may be observed, accompanied by a structural and biochemical remodeling of the ECM, including 1) perivascular and interstitial fibrosis, and 2) increased thickness of perimysial tendons, weave and strands. An increment in systolic and diastolic stress-strain relations caused by an increased collagen volume fraction in hypertrophic myocardium is clinically expressed as diastolic left ventricular dysfunction with a preservation of systolic function.[62] What modulates the appearance of this fibrous tissue? Development of left ventricular hypertrophy has been observed in every rat model of arterial hypertension, but the fibrous tissue response occurred only when the renin-angiotensin-aldosteron system was activated or when circulating mineralocorticoid levels were elevated.[63] Furthermore, myocardial fibrosis was observed in both ventricles, despite the fact that the right ventricle was not overloaded and, therefore, not hypertrophied. Treatment of spontaneously hypertensive rats (having left ventricular hypertrophy) with low dose (2.5 mg/kg/day) and high dose (20 mg/kg/day) lisinopril for 12 weeks, starting at an age of 14 weeks, blocked the fibrous tissue response, independent of lowering of blood pressure and regression of left ventricular hypertrophy.[64]

Conclusions

The interaction between myocardial overload and biological effects in the myocardium is accomplished by physical factors that are relayed to the interior of the cells by mechano-chemical coupling. Likely candidates are 1) mechano-sensitive membrane proteins, including ion channels and ion exchangers, 2) stretch-induced release of growth factors, hormones and cytokines, and 3) integrin receptor stimulation. These candidate couplers of overload to biological effects may be active at specific stages of development of hypertrophy. Paracrine interaction between cells and cell types through release of growth-stimulating factors complicates the scheme of events leading to hypertrophy. However, the wealth of growth-inducing factors and conditions and their specific role in (a certain stage of) developing hypertrophy may explain why the resulting hypertrophic phenotype strongly depends on the stimulus that caused hypertrophy.

References

1. Bustamante JO, Ruknudin A, Sachs F. Stretch-activated channels in heart cells: relevance to cardiac hypertrophy. J Cardiovasc Pharmacol 1991;17:S110-S3.

2. Sigurdson W, Ruknudin A, Sachs F. Calcium imaging of mechanically induced fluxes in tissue-cultured chick heart: role of stretch-activated ion channels. Am J Physiol 1992;262:H1110-H5.

3. Sadoshima J, Takahashi T, Jahn L, Izumo S. Role of mechanosensitive ion channels, cytoskeleton, and contractile activity in stretch-induced immediate-early gene expression and hypertrophy of cardiac myocytes. Proc Natl Acad Sci USA 1992;89:9905-9.

4. Yamazaki T, Komuro I, Kudoh S, et al. Role of ion channels and exchangers in mechanical stretch-induced cardiomyocyte hypertrophy. Circ Res 1998;82:430-7.

5. Molkentin JD, Lu JR, Antos CL, et al. A calcineurin-dependent transcriptional pathway for cardiac hypertrophy. Cell 1998;93:215-28.

6. Shadoshima J, Izumo S. Mechanical stretch rapidly activates multiple signal transduction pathways in cardiac myocytes: potential involvement of an autocrine/paracrine mechanism. EMBO J 1993;12:1681-92.

7. von Harsdorf R, Lang RE, Fullerton M, Woodcock EA. Myocardial stretch stimulates phosphatidylinositol turnover. Circ Res 1989;65:494-501.

8. Kaye D, Pimental D, Prasad S, et al. Role of transiently altered sarcolemmal membrane permeability and basic fibroblast growth factor release in the hypertrophic response of adult rat ventricular myocytes to increased mechanical activity in vitro. J Clin Invest 1996;97:281-91.

9. Clarke MSF, Caldwell RW, Chiao H, Miyake K, McNeil PL. Contraction-induced cell wounding and release of fibroblast growth factor in heart. Circ Res 1995;76:927-34.

10. Schaub MC, Hefti MA, Harder BA, Eppenberger HM. Various hypertrophic stimuli induce distinct phenotypes in cardiomyocytes. J Mol Med 1997;75:901-20.

11. Parker TG, Packer SE, Schneider MD. Peptide growth factors can provojke "fetal" contractile protein gene expression in rat cardiac myocytes. J Clin Invest 1990;85:507-14.

12. Parker TG, Chow KL, Schwartz RJ, Schneider MD. Differential regulation of skeletal alpha-actin transcription in cardiac muscle by two fibroblast growth factors. Proc Natl Acad Sci USA 1990;87:7066-70.

13. Villareal FJ, Dillmann WH. Cardiac hypertrophy-induced changes in mRNA levels for TGF-ß$_1$, fibronectin, and collagen. Am J Physiol 1992;262:H1861-H6.

14. Takahashi N, Calderone A, Izzo NJ jr, Mäki TM, Marsh JD, Colucci WS. Hypertrophic stimuli induce transforming growth factor-ß$_1$ expression in rat ventricular myocytes. J Clin Invest 1994;94:1470-6.

15. Calderone A, Takahashi N, Izzo NJ jr, Thaik CM, Colucci WS. Pressure- and volume-induced left ventricular hypertrophies are associated with distinct myocyte phenotypes and differential induction of peptide growth factor mRNAs. Circulation 1995;92:2385-90.

16. Eghbali M. Cellular origin and distribution of transforming growth factor-ß$_1$ in the normal rat myocardium. Cell Tissue Res 1989;256:553-8.

17. Parker TG, Chow KL, Schwartz RJ, Schneider MD. TGFß$_1$ and fibroblast growth factors selectively upregulate tissue-specific fetal genes in cardiac muscle cells. Ciba Found Symp 1991;157:152-64.

18. Long CS. Autocrine and paracrine regulation of myocardial cell growth in vitro. The TGFß paradigm. Trends Cardiovasc Med 1996;6:217-26.

19. Shubeita HE, McDonough PM, Harris AN, et al. Endothelin induction of inositol phospholipid hydrolysis, sarcomere assembly, and cardiac gene expression in ventricular myocytes. J Biol Chem 1990;265:20555-62.

20. Neyses L, Nouskas J, Vetter H. Inhibition of endothelin-1 induced myocardial protein synthesis by an antisense oligonucleotide against early growth response gene-1. Biochem Biophys Res Comm 1991;181:22-7.

21. Ito H, Hirata Y, Hiroe M, et al. Endothelin-1 induces hypertrophy with enhanced expression of muscle-specific genes in cultured neonatal rat cardiomyocytes. Circ Res 1991;69:209-15.

22. Ito H, Hiroe M, Hirata Y, et al. Endothelin ET$_A$ receptor antagonist blocks cardiac hypertrophy provoked by hemodynamic overload. Circulation 1994;89:2198-203.

23. Suzuki T, Tsuruda A, Katoh S, Kubodera A, Mitsui Y. Purification of endothelin from a conditioned medium od cardiac fibroblastic cells using beating rate assay of myocytes cultured in a serum-free medium. J Mol Cell Cardiol 1997;29:2087-93.

24. Harada M, Itoh H, Nakagawa O, et al. Significance of ventricular myocytes and nonmyocytes interaction during cardiac hypertrophy. Evidence for endothelin-1 as a pracrine hypertrophic factor from cardiac nonmyocytes. Circulation 1997;96:3737-44.

25. Sadoshima JI, Xu Y, Slayter HS, Izumo S. Autocrine release of angiotensin II mediates tretch-induced hypertrophy of cardiac myocytes in vitro. Cell 1993;75:977-84.

26. Sadoshima J, Izumo S. Molecular characterization of angiotensin II-induced hypertrophy of cardiac

myocytes and hyperplasia of cardiac fibroblasts: critical role for the AT1-receptor subtype. Circ Res 1993;73:413-23.

27.   Linz W, Schoelkens BA, Ganten D. Converting enzyme inhibitor specifically prevents development and induces the regression of cardiac hypertrophy in rats. Clin Exp Hypertens A 1989;11:1325-50.

28.   Linz W, Schaper J, Wiemer G, Albus U, Scholkens BA. Ramipril prevents left ventricular hypertrophy with myocardial fibrosis without blood pressure reduction: a one year study in rats. Br J Pharmacol 1992;107:970-5.

29.   Kim NN, Villarreal FJ, Printz MP, Lee AA, Dillmann WH. Trophic effects of angiotensin II on neonatal rat cardiac myocytes are mediated by cardiac fibroblasts. Am J Physiol 1995;269:E426-E437.

30.   Ponicke K, Heinroth-Hoffmann I, Becker K, Brodde OE. Trophic effect of angiotensin II in neonatal rat cardiomyocytes: role of endothelin-1 and non-myocyte cells. Br J Pharmacol 1997;121:118-24.

31.   Gray MO, Long CS, Kalinyak JE, Li HT, Karliner JS. Angiotensin II stimulates cardiac myocyte hypertrophy via paracrine release of TGF-β_1 and endothelin-1 from fibroblasts. Cardiovasc Res 1998;40:352-63.

32.   Chen CS, Mrksich M, Huang S, Whitesides GM, Ingber DE. Geometric control of cell life and death. Science 1997;276:1425-8.

33.   Wang N, Butler JP, Ingber DE. Mechanotransduction across the cell surface and through the cytoskeleton. Science 1993;260:1124-7.

34.   Tsutsui H, Ishihara K, Cooper G. Cytoskeletal role in the contractile dysfunction of hypertrophied myocardium. Science 1993;260:682-7.

35.   Collins JF, Pawloski-Dahm C, Davis MG, Ball N, Dorn GW, Walsh RA. The role of the cytoskeleton in left ventricular pressure overload hypertrophy and failure. J Mol Cell Cardiol 1996;28:1435-43.

36.   Sato H, Nagai T, Kuppuswamy D, et al. Microtubule stabilization in pressure overload cardiac hypertrophy. J Cell Biol 1997;139:963-73.

37.   Katz AM. The cardiomyopathy of overload: an unnatural growth response. Eur Heart J 1995;16 (Suppl O):110-4.

38.   Moalic JM, Charlemagne D, Mansier P, Chevalier B, Swynghedauw B. Cardiac hypertrophy and failure - A disease of adaptation. Modifications in membrane proteins provide a molecular basis for arrhythmogenicity. Circulation 1993;87(Suppl IV):IV21-IV26.

39.   Vliegen HW, Van der Laarse A, Cornelisse CJ, Eulderink F. Myocardial changes in pressure overload-induced left ventricular hypertrophy. A study on tissue composition, polyploidization and multinucleation. Eur Heart J 1991;12:488-94.

40.   Van Wamel AJET, Ruwhof C, Van der Valk LJM, Schrier PI, Van der Laarse A. Paracrine effects of stretch on expression of immediate-early genes and atrial natriuretic peptide in cardiomyocytes [abstract]. Eur Heart J 1998;19(abstr suppl):37.

41.   McKenna DA, Dolfi F, Vuori K, Ruoslahti E. Extracellular signal-regulated kinase and c-Jun NH_2-terminal kinase activation by mechanical stretch is integrin-dependent and matrix-specific in rat cardiac fibroblasts. J Clin Invest 1998;101:301-10.

42.   Predel HG, Yang Z, Von Segesser L, Turina M, Bühler FR, Lüscher TF. Implications of pulsatile stretch on growth of saphenous vein and mammary artery smooth muscle. Lancet 1992;340:878-9.

43.   Yang Z, Noll G, Lüscher TF. Calcium antagonists inhibit proliferation of human coronary smooth muscle cells in response to pulsatile stretch and platelet-derived growth factor. Circulation 1993;88:832-6.

44.   Hishikawa K, Oemar BS, Yang Z, Lüscher TF. Pulsatile stretch stimulates superoxide production and activates nuclear factor- B in human coronary smooth muscle. Circ Res 1997;81:797-803.

45.   Li G, Mills I, Sumpio BE. Cyclic strain stimulates endothelial cell proliferation: characterization of strain requirements. Endothelium 1994;2:177-81.

46.   Iba T, Sumpio BE. Tissue plasminogen activator expression in endothelial cells exposed to cyclic strain in vitro. Cell Transplant 1992;1:43-50.

47.   Awolesi MA, Sessa WC, Sumpio BE. Cyclic strain upregulates nitric oxide synthase in cultured bovine aortic endothelial cells. J Clin Invest 1995;96:1449-54.

48.   Awolesi MA, Widmann MD, Sessa WC, Sumpio BE. Cyclic strain increases endothelial nitric oxide synthase activity. Surgery 1994;116:439-45.

49.   Wang DL, Wung BS, Shyy YD, et al. Mechanical strain induces monocyte chemotactic protein-1 gene expression in endothelial cells. Effects of mechanical strain on monocyte adhesion to endothelial cells. Circ Res 1995;77:294-302.

50.   Regulation of PDGF-B in endothelial cells exposed to cyclic strain. Sumpio BE, Du W, Galagher G, et al. Arterioscler Thromb Vasc Biol 1998;18:349-55.

51.   Carroll SM, Nimmo LE, Knoepfler PS, White FC, Bloor CM. Gene expression in a swine model of right ventricular hypertrophy: intercellular adhesion molecule, vascular endothelial growth factor and plasminogen activators are upregulated during pressure overload. J Mol Cell Cardiol 1995;27:1427-41.

52. Wang DL, Wung BS, Peng YC, Wang JJ. Mechanical strain increases endothelin-1 gene expression via protein kinase C pathway in human endothelial cells. J Cell Physiol 1995;163:400-6.
53. Wang DL, Tang CC, Wung BS, Chen HH, Hung MS, Wang JJ. Cyclical strain increases endothelin-1 secretion and gene expression in human endothelial cells. Biochem Biophys Res Comm 1993;195:1050-6.
54. Li J, Hampton T, Morgan JP, Simons M. Stretch-induced VEGF expression in the heart. J Clin Invest 1997;100:18-24.
55. Schaper W. Control of coronary angiogenesis. Eur Heart J 1995;16(Suppl C):66-8.
56. Breisch EA, Houser SR, Carey RA, Spann JF, Bove AA. Myocardial blood flow and capillary density in chronic pressure overload of the feline left ventricle. Cardiovasc Res 1980;14:469-75.
57. Rakusan K, Flanagan MF, Geva T, Southern J, Vanpraagh R. Morphometry of human coronary capillaries during normal growth and the effect of age in left ventricular pressure -overload hypertrophy. Circulation 1992;86:38-46.
58. Tomanek RJ. Response of the coronary vasculature to myocardial hypertrophy. J Am Coll Cardiol 1990;15:528-33.
59. Tomanek RJ, Palmer PJ, Pfeiffer GL, Schreiber KL, Eastham CL, Marcus ML. Morphometry of canine coronary arteries, arterioles and capillaries during hypertension and left ventricular hypertrophy. Circ Res 1986;58:38-46.
60. Tomanek RJ, Torry RJ. Growth of the coronary vasculature in hypertrophy; mechanisms and model dependence. Cell Mol Biol Res 1994;40:129-36.
61. Hudlicka O, Brown MD. Postnatal growth of the heart and its blood vessels. J Vasc Res 1996;33:266-87.
62. Weber KT. Cardiac interstitium in health and disease: the fibrillar collagen network. J Am Coll Cardiol 1989;13:1637-52.
63. Brilla CG, Pick R, Tan LB, Janicki JS, Weber KT. Remodeling of the rat right and left ventricle in experimental hypertension. Circ Res 1990;67:1355-64.
64. Brilla CG, Janicki JS, Weber KT. Impaired diastolic function and coronary reserve in genetic hypertension: role of interstitial fibrosis and medial thickening of intramyocardial coronary arteries. Circ Res 1991;69:107-15

2. THE ROLE OF VASCULAR FAILURE IN HEART FAILURE

R.A. TIO, R. DE BOER, D.J. VAN VELDHUISEN, W.H. VAN GILST

Summary

Next to important adaptation mechanisms such as changes in the autonomic nervous system and humoral systems (e.g. the renin-angiotensin system), changes in the vascular wall play an important role in heart failure. The normal endothelium dependent, nitric oxide (NO) mediated vasodilative function is lost in heart failure. The impaired NO capacity may add to reduced tissue perfusion as well as a reduced angiogenic potential. From this the hypothesis evolves that impaired "endothelial function" may lead to ischemia and further deterioration of left ventricular function. Treatment strategies aimed at a better endothelial function and angiogenesis seem therefore promising in retarding progression of heart failure.

Introduction

Heart failure is defined as the inability of the heart to supply peripheral tissues with an adequate perfusion. It is a leading cause of morbidity and mortality in the developed world. The reported survival rates range between 48% and 79% at 1 year.[1] Repeat hospitalizations due to exacerbations are fairly common. Concomitantly, the health care costs pose us with an increasing economic burden.[2]

The most common cause of heart failure is ischemic heart disease. The initial event lies in a reduction of left ventricular pump function. In the past, the reduced pump function and systemic adaptation mechanisms, in particular autonomic and humoral changes have been focused on. The heart in this view can be considered as cause and central player in the further deterioration of left ventricular function. In this chapter we will focus on the role of peripheral, i.e. vascular changes that play a pivotal role, and the relation with neurohumoral changes, in the further deterioration of left ventricular function.

E. E. van der Wall et al.(eds.), Left Ventricular Hypertrophy, 15-20.
© 1999 *Kluwer Academic Publishers. Printed in the Netherlands.*

In chronic heart failure initial systemic adaptation mechanisms are aimed at maintenance of an adequate blood pressure to face the reduced cardiac output.[3] Alterations in the autonomic nervous system result in increased sympathetic and decreased parasympathetic tone. Initially this will cause a higher heart rate and contractility, and peripheral vasoconstriction. As a result cardiac output and a blood pressure are increased. Eventually the chronically increased sympathetic tone will become less effective because of ∃-receptor down regulation and desensitization. Furthermore, the increased sympathetic tone has also been associated with adverse cardiac events, such as lethal ventricular rhythm disturbances.[4]

Activation of the renin angiotensin system (RAS) results in fluid retention (aldosteron effect) and more importantly myocardial (and vascular) hypertrophy (angiotensin-II effect).[5] Angiotensin-II is a potent growth factor resulting in the heart, in myocyte hypertrophy and non-myocyte proliferation and intercellular matrix formation. Its effect on blood vessels is, apart from vasoconstriction, induction of vascular smooth muscle cell proliferation.

Vascular failure

Although both mentioned adaptation mechanisms cause peripheral vasoconstriction, regulation of the vascular tone is also disturbed in the vessel wall itself.[6] The term vascular failure, or more appropriately endothelial failure or dysfunction has been introduced for this phenomenon. Normal arteries contain an endothelial cell layer that is capable of producing various vasoactive substances. Nitric oxide is the most prominent vasodilating substance produced by the endothelium. Next to vasodilatation, it reduces platelet aggregation, leukocyte adhesion, and vascular smooth muscle cell proliferation, and it plays a role in angiogenesis.[6] The vasodilating properties of endothelium derived NO can relatively easy be assessed in vivo in humans. By means of an agonist such as acetylcholine that stimulates NO release from the endothelium, endothelium dependent vasodilatation can be assessed in coronary as well as peripheral arteries. In case of an inadequate NO release the artery will not dilate or even constrict due to the direct effect of acetylcholine on the vascular smooth muscle cells.[7]

A reduced endothelium dependent relaxation has been found in patients with heart failure, in coronary as well as peripheral arteries. This might be due to a decreased NO production. Expression of endothelial NO synthase is reduced in experimental heart failure [6] On the other hand, an increased NO breakdown may also be involved. There is evidence that heart failure is associated with increased oxidative stress.[8] The associated free radicals may react with the endothelium derived NO. In this manner the biological activity of the NO will be diminished. This might explain the finding that vitamin C may improve endothelium dependent vasomotor activity.[9]

Ischemia hypothesis

Physiological enlargement during normal development and growth and in response to intense exercise is characterized by an equal increase in both compartments. Physiologic adaptation of the heart such as after the transition from the prenatal to the postnatal workload situation, is achieved by hypertrophy of the cardiomyocytes, i.e. cardiomyocytes increase in length as well as in diameter. Simultaneously, the number of mitochondria and contractile myofibrils per cell increases. In order to meet the increased metabolic demand of the increased myocyte mass new capillaries are formed as well.[10]

In contrast, myocardial adaptation in response to overload after myocardial infarction, characteristically disturbs normal myocardial architecture, resulting in a relative increase of extracellular matrix and a decrease in capillary density.[10,11] The relative deficit of capillaries in turn may leave the hypertrophied myocardium more susceptible to ischemia.

Angiogenesis, sprouting of new capillaries from the pre-existing vascular network rarely occurs in the heart under normal conditions. Endothelial cells play a pivotal role in angiogenesis.[12] Endothelial cells respond to angiogenic stimuli by initiating the formation of new vessels. In this process endothelial cells produce metalloproteinases to digest the basement membrane, then they can break loose from the basement membrane, migrate, proliferate and form a network of endothelial tubes. Subsequently, other cells (pericytes) will surround these endothelial tubes to form the primordial vessels.

The renin-angiotensin system (RAS) is being considered as one of the most important regulatory systems for cardiovascular homeostasis. It plays a central role in blood pressure regulation, and in growth processes in the vessel wall as well as the myocardium.[13] The beneficial effects of angiotensin converting enzyme (ACE)-inhibitors on hypertrophied myocardium have been described extensively in animal and in human studies.[13] ACE-inhibitors not only reduce symptoms, but also improve survival in heart failure patients.[13] Despite these beneficial effects systemic treatment with ACE-inhibitors and possibly AT1-receptor antagonists does not prevent further deterioration of left ventricular function.

Treatment aimed at improved tissue perfusion

Treatment with ACE-inhibitors in patients after a myocardial infarction and reduced left ventricular function prevented further ischemic cardiac events in the SOLVD [14] and the SAVE[15] trials. In the CATS study, it was found that this reduction in ischemic events appeared to develop as early as 3 months after myocardial infarction.[16] The effects of ACE-inhibitors on endothelial function add to the beneficial effects in heart failure. It has been shown that treatment with ACE-inhibitors improves endothelial function in a wide variety of models and situations. In experimental studies ACE-inhibition resulted in a bradykinin dependent release of NO and prostacyclin. In patients with coronary artery disease an impaired endothelium dependent relaxation is often present. When such patients were treated with quinapril or placebo, the initial vasoconstrictive response was significantly reduced towards a vasodilating response in the quinapril group. No such improvement was found in the placebo group.[17]

Given all the above, it is not surprising that activation of the RAS as found after myocardial infarction contributes to unfavorable remodeling of the myocardium: cardiomyocyte hypertrophy, increased matrix deposition, and relative deficit of neo-vascularisation or angiogenesis, next to increased afterload and neurohumoral activation. Interference with the ACE (Angiotensin-II formation and bradykinin breakdown) may therefore have a dual synergistic effect: reduction of hypertrophy and extra-cellular matrix formation on one hand, and angiogenesis on the other hand. It seems promising, therefore, to further identify how components of the RAS can be optimally regulated with regard to these specific actions.

Next to ACE-inhibitors many other pharmacological agents have been shown to improve endothelium dependent relaxation. Interestingly, new pharmacological interventions, physical training programs are also associated with improvement in endothelium. After a physical training protocol in one extremity, flow induced endothelium dependent vasodilatation was improved in the trained extremity only.[18] One explanation may be that local mechanical forces such as the increased shear stress play a pivotal role in this process. Shear stress can induce expression of endothelial NO synthase,[19] causing an improved endothelium dependent relaxation. Physical training has been shown to increase eNOS expression in aortic endothelium in dogs. Preservation of endothelium dependent vasodilatation was associated with improved resting hemodynamics and diminished heart failure symptoms in this model.[20] In addition to shear stress mediated upregulation of eNOS expression, shear stress may also downregulate the expression of ACE.[21] This by itself may improve endothelium dependent vasodilatation, by increased bradykinin concentrations. Bradykinin is a potent stimulus for NO release from the endothelium.

Another explanation by which physical training improves endothelium dependent vasodilatation may be due to ischemia. The exercise will induce tissue ischemia. Ischemia is a strong stimulus for upregulation of vascular endothelial growth factor (VEGF) expression.[22] VEFG in turn can not only upregulate eNOS expression [23] but also accelerate endothelial regeneration and induce angiogenesis.[24] All these functions of VEGF will result in an improved tissue perfusion.

Conclusions

In this chapter we discussed the neurohumoral changes in relation to endothelial dysfunction in heart failure. Especially, a reduced capacity of the endothelium to produce NO may add to further deterioration of tissue perfusion and left ventricular function. Strategies to improve NO production include ACE-inhibition and exercise. These two strategies both aim at maintenance or improvement of (peripheral as well as myocardial) tissue perfusion. Finally, the same problem of relative underperfusion and subsequent ischemia may play a pivotal role in the further deterioration of left ventricular function. Therefore, improvement in endothelial function and induction of angiogenesis seem to be a promising strategy.

References

1. Cowie MR, Mosterd A, Wood DA, et al. The epidemiology of heart failure. Eur Heart J 1997;18:208-25.
2. Hoes AW, Mosterd A, Grobbee DE. An epidemic of heart failure? Recent evidence from Europe. Eur Heart J 1998;19 Suppl L:L2-9.
3. Zelis R, Flaim SF. Alterations in vasomotor tone in congestive heart failure. Prog Cardiovasc Dis 1982;24:437-59.
4. Cohn JN, Levine TB, Olivari MT, et al. Plasma norepinephrine as a guide to prognosis in patients with chronic congestive heart failure. N Engl J Med 1984;311:819-23.
5. Pitt B. ACE inhibitors in heart failure: prospects and limitations. Cardiovasc Drugs Ther 1997;11 Suppl 1:285-90.
6. Smith CJ, Sun D, Hoegler C, et al. Reduced gene expression of vascular endothelial NO synthase and cyclooxygenase-1 in heart failure. Circ Res 1996;78:58-64.
7. Furchgott RF, Zawadzki JV. The obligatory role of endothelial cells in the relaxation of arterial smooth muscle by acetylcholine. Nature 1980;288:373-6.
8. Belch JJ, Bridges AB, Scott N, Chopra M. Oxygen free radicals and congestive heart failure. Br Heart J;65:245-8.
9. Hornig B, Arakawa N, Kohler C, Drexler H. Vitamin C improves endothelial function of conduit arteries in patients with chronic heart failure. Circulation 1998;97:363-8.
10. Aversa P, Ricci R, Olivetti G. Quantitative structural analysis of the myocardium during physiologic growth and induced cardiac hypertrophy: a review. J Am Coll Cardiol 1986;7:1140-9.
11. Weber KT. Cardiac interstitium in health and disease: the fibrillar collagen network. J Am Coll Cardiol 1989;13:1637-52.
12. Isner JM. Vascular endothelial growth factor: gene therapy and therapeutic angiogenesis. Am J Cardiol 1998;82:63S-64S.
13. Brown NJ, Vaughan DE. Angiotensin-converting enzyme inhibitors. Circulation 1998;97:1411-2.
14. Yusuf S, Pepine CJ, Garces C, et al. Effect of enalapril on myocardial infarction and unstable angina in patients with low ejection fractions. Lancet 1992;340:1173-8.
15. Pfeffer MA, Braunwald E, Moye LA, et al. Effect of captopril on mortality and morbidity in patients with left ventricular dysfunction after myocardial infarction. Results of the survival and ventricular enlargement trial. The SAVE Investigators. N Engl J Med 1992;327:669-77.
16. Van den Heuvel F, Van Gilst WH, Van Veldhuisen DJ, De Vries RJ, Dunselman PH, Kingma JH. Long-term anti-ischemic effects of angiotensin-converting enzyme inhibition in patients after myocardial infarction. The Captopril and Thrombolysis Study (CATS) Investigators. J Am Coll Cardiol 1997;30:400-5.
17. Mancini GBJ, Henry GC, Macaya C, et al. Angiotensin-converting enzyme inhibition with quinapril improves endothelial vasomotor dysfunction in patients with coronary artery disease. The TREND (Trial on Reversing ENdothelial Dysfunction) Study. Circulation 1996;94:258-65.
18. Hornig B, Maier V, Drexler H. Physical training improves endothelial function in patients with chronic heart failure. Circulation 1996;93:210-4.
19. Nishida K, Harrison DG, Navas JP, et al. Molecular cloning and characterization of the constitutive bovine aortic endothelial cell nitric oxide synthase. J Clin Invest 1992;90:2092-6.
20. Wang J, Yi GH, Knecht M, et al. Physical training alters the pathogenesis of pacing-induced heart failure through endothelium-mediated mechanisms in awake dogs. Circulation 1997;96:2683-92.
21. Rieder MJ, Carmona R, Krieger JE, Pritchard KAJ, Greene AS. Suppression of angiotensin-converting enzyme expression and activity by shear stress. Circ Res 1997;80:312-9.
22. Namiki A, Brogi E, Kearney M, Kim EA, Wu T, Couffinhal T, et al. Hypoxia induces vascular endothelial growth factor in cultured human endothelial cells. J Biol Chem 1995;270:31189-95.
23. Kroll J, Waltenberger J. VEGF-A induces expression of eNOS and iNOS in endothelial cells via VEGF receptor-2 (KDR). Biochem.Biophys Res Commun 1998;252:743-6.
24. Asahara T, Chen D, Tsurumi Y, et al. Accelerated restitution of endothelial integrity and endothelium-dependent function after phVEGF165 gene transfer. Circulation 1996;94:3291-302.

3. PERFUSION ABNORMALITIES IN THE HYPERTROPHIED LEFT VENTRICLE: LINK BETWEEN COMPENSATED HYPERTROPHY AND HEART FAILURE?

D.J.G.M. DUNCKER

Introduction

Cardiac hypertrophy occurs in a variety of conditions and serves to normalize elevated levels of systolic wall stress. Thus, increased afterload due to increased impedance to left ventricular outflow or hypertension (pressure-overload), increased preload to accommodate an increased stroke volume (volume-overload) or loss of contractile tissue (myocardial infarction) all produce an increase in cardiac mass. Although initially appropriate, myocardial hypertrophy has been shown to be an independent risk factor for the development of heart failure (i.e. independent of the underlying cause of hypertrophy),[1] suggesting that hypertrophy itself and not only the underlying disease puts the heart at risk of progressing into a state of overt pumping failure. The transition from compensated hypertrophy to overt heart failure, is still incompletely understood, but must result from either myocardial (cardiomyocyte or the extracellular matrix) or coronary factors (altered myocardial perfusion). In this chapter, characteristics and underlying mechanisms of systolic and diastolic dysfunction of the pressure-overloaded hypertrophied left ventricle will be discussed, in particular the potential role of altered myocardial perfusion in the progression from compensated (i.e. normal global systolic function) to decompensated hypertrophic remodeling. Since systemic hypertension is one of the major causes for left ventricular hypertrophy, and since this is usually associated with a prolonged period of compensated hypertrophy, focus will be on the characteristics of hypertrophy produced by pressure-overload.

E. E. van der Wall et al.(eds.), Left Ventricular Hypertrophy, 21-41.
© 1999 *Kluwer Academic Publishers. Printed in the Netherlands.*

Systolic function in the hypertrophied heart

There is general agreement that at least during the early development of hypertrophy process left ventricular systolic contractile function is normal in the pressure-overload hypertrophied heart (hence the term "compensated hypertrophy"), as indicated by the normal systolic wall stress and the normal ejection fraction. Normal systolic contractile function is also indicated by contractility indices in-vivo,[2] such as a normal maximum rate of rise of left ventricular pressure (LVdP/dt$_{max}$), and by isotonic and isometric indices, such as maximum tension, in isolated papillary muscle in-vitro.[3,4] These studies also indicate that contractile reserve in response to inotropic stimulation is well preserved.[2-4] There are a number of studies that report depressed peak tension in, particularly severely, hypertrophied left ventricles, but it is difficult to exclude that these hearts have not already begun the transition from compensated hypertrophy to heart failure.[5] This is corroborated by studies that find only a decrease in contractility and calcium transients of individual cardiomyocytes when there are signs of heart failure.[6,7] Moreover, even when global left ventricular systolic performance is normal this does not necessarily mean that the contraction pattern is also completely normal, as hypertrophied myocardium is characterized by a lower maximum velocity of contraction (V$_{max}$) (Figure 1).[8-10] This shift towards a slower contraction may occur to allow an energetically more favorable contraction pattern as the slower contraction is associated with an increased economy (ratio of tension-time integral and oxygen cost) and efficiency (ratio of work and oxygen cost) of contraction in the face of an increase in load.[9]

What is the mechanism for the slower contraction? The mechanism for the slower contraction could be either a slower calcium transient or an alteration in the responsiveness of the myofilaments to calcium. While in rats a shift from the V$_1$ to V$_3$ myosin heavy chain isoform plays an important role in slowing contraction during the development of left ventricular hypertrophy,[10-12] owing to the lower myosin ATP-ase activity and thus slower turnover rate of cross-bridge cycling, the V$_3$ isoform is already native to adult myocardium of large animals and humans. Although there are a number of other changes in the sarcomeres, for example the reappearance of atrial myosin light chains in the ventricles,[13,14] the implications of these changes for contractile performance of the hypertrophied left ventricle are still not fully clear.[10-14] Hence, alterations in calcium transients are currently

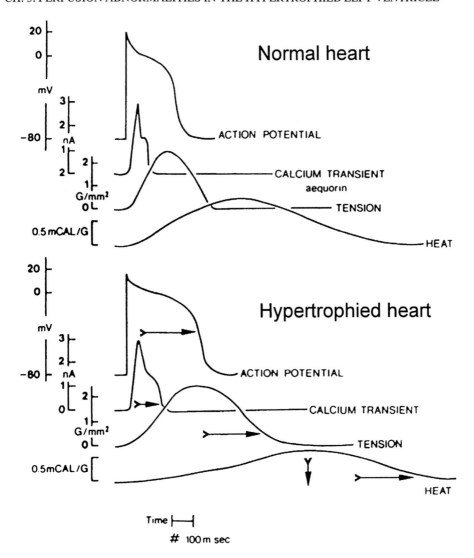

Figure 1. Excitation-contraction coupling and heat production in the hypertrophied heart compared with the normal heart. In the hypertrophied heart, the calcium transient measured by aequorin is prolonged and the contraction and relaxation are both prolonged.[8] It is proposed that the hypertrophied heart works more economically, which can be seen from the reduced rate of heat production.[9] (From Swynghedauw et al.[10], with permission).

considered to be the predominant underlying cause for the slower contraction (Figure 1).

Indeed, several studies have shown that the calcium transients are slower in hypertrophied

myocardium. In contrast, the peak calcium concentration is normal[8] which may explain why inotropic responses to calcium and calcium agonists are normal.[15] The mechanism for the slowing of calcium transients in hypertrophied myocardium is still incompletely understood, but there is ample evidence that calcium removal is slowed in the hypertrophied cardiomyocyte (see below). In addition, the function of calcium release channels in the sarcoplasmic reticulum may be impaired due to a decreased density of the ryanodine receptors that regulate their activity.[16] Observations that the action potential duration is prolonged (due to alterations in the transient outward current) point towards a prolonged transarcolemmal calcium influx (during the prolonged plateau phase) which could serve to compensate for a decreased sarcolemmal calcium channel density as has been reported in severe hypertrophy.[17] Although the density of dihydropyridine binding receptors per cell surface area is unchanged in moderately hypertrophied left ventricular cardiomyocytes,[11] it is still possible (since volume is related to the third power of the radius and surface area is related to the second power of the radius), that even during moderate hypertrophy a relative decrease in "volume density" of sarcolemmal channels occurs. A recent study reported normal transsarcolemmal calcium influx and normal sarcoplasmic calcium release channel function. To account for a slowing of the calcium channels, the authors proposed that as a consequence of the increased cell size a change in the spatial relation between the sarcolemmal and sarcoplasmic calcium channels could have occurred, thereby blunting the ability of the transsarcolemmal activator calcium to trigger sarcoplasmic calcium release.[18]

Diastolic function in the hypertrophied heart

In contrast to the maintained systolic contractile performance of the hypertrophied left ventricle well into the later stages of the hypertrophy process, much earlier in the process of hypertrophic remodeling the left ventricle is characterized by an increased diastolic chamber stiffness. An increase in chamber stiffness (dP/dV) can occur simply as a result of an increase in operating volume stiffness without a change in the modulus of chamber stiffness (Kp_{LV}), but can also result from an increased Kp_{LV} (Figure 2).[19] The latter can be due to either an increased left ventricular wall thickness (in the presence of a normal myocardial stiffness, Kp_M), or to an increase in Kp_M secondary to quantitative and qualitative changes in myocardial collagen content. In the hypertrophied heart, collagen

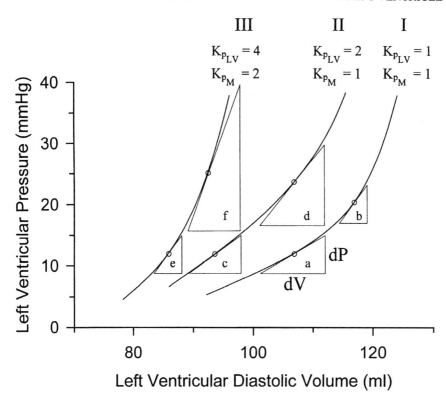

Figure 2. Left ventricular diastolic pressure-volume relations. Situation I denotes a normal left ventricle with chamber and myocardial stiffness constants set arbitrarily at 1. An increase in chamber stiffness can occur due to an increase in operating volume stiffness without changes in chamber stiffness modulus ($K_{p\,LV} = 1$) or myocardial stiffness modulus ($K_{p\,M} = 1$), when diastolic volume increases (from situation Ia to Ib). When hypertrophy occurs (a thicker wall in the absence of altered myocardial material properties) an increase in chamber stiffness occurs due an increase in chamber stiffness modulus ($K_{p\,LV} = 2$) but without an increase in myocardial stiffness ($K_{p\,M} = 1$), which is depicted in situations IIc and IId. When material properties eventually change (e.g. due to fibrosis) the chamber stiffness can increase further resulting from the increase in myocardial stiffness modulus ($K_{p\,M} = 2$) that in turn increases the chamber stiffness modulus ($K_{p\,LV} = 4$), which is depicted in situations IIIe and IIIf. (Based on Gaasch et al[19] and Weber et al[20]).

composition appears to be minimally affected so that changes in myocardial stiffness are most likely due to alterations in collagen concentration. Weber and colleagues have described 3 types of myocardial fibrosis responses in the hypertrophied heart.[20] The first is a reactive fibrosis in which collagen concentration is not changed but collagen is deposited in keeping with the increased muscle mass. In this situation muscle stiffness would not be expected to be increased. Fibrosis is called excessive when collagen fibers become thicker, surrounding and even choking, the myocytes. In this situation muscle stiffness will increase. In later stages, restorative fibrosis is added to the reactive type to fill up centers of necrosis, with collagen fibers running perpendicular to the muscle fibers resulting in large increments in stiffness. Finally, the hypertrophied left ventricle is characterized by an impairment of relaxation resulting in a slower decay of myocardial elastance or active myocardial stiffness. Thus, the prolonged and slowed calcium transient is characterized not only by a decreased velocity of contraction but also by a slowing of relaxation which is most likely due to a decrease in relative sarcoplasmic calcium ATP-ase content.[21,22]

Implications of diastolic dysfunction. The early diastolic functional abnormalities do not appear to have an adverse effect on resting systolic pump function, as the latter may continue to be normal for a prolonged period of time.[11,13] During exercise the relaxation abnormalities could potentially result in a compromised pump function due to a reduced effective diastolic filling time, requiring marked increases in left ventricular filling pressures to maintain preload and hence stroke volume. However, the effect of diastolic function on myocardial perfusion appears to be more important. First, a slowing of relaxation will result in blunting of the typically steep rise in coronary blood flow during early diastole, thereby impeding early diastolic perfusion. This will predominantly affect the subendocardial layers since these are almost exclusively perfused during diastole. Second, an increase in passive stiffness (increased wall thickness and increased collagen content) requires higher diastolic pressures in order to attain the appropriate end-diastolic volume, and thereby increase diastolic radial wall stress which also acts to impede coronary blood flow.

Perfusion abnormalities in the hypertrophied left ventricle

There is overwhelming evidence that the compensated hypertrophied heart is characterized by an increased susceptibility to subendocardial ischemia. Thus, in patients with angiographically normal epicardial coronary arteries, exercise was associated with angina pectoris[23] and electrocardiographic changes suggestive of subendocardial ischemia.[24] In addition, post-mortem studies demonstrated increased subendocardial fibrosis and papillary infarction in patients with left ventricular hypertrophy and normal coronary arteries.[23,25]

Similarly, in dogs with severe left ventricular hypertrophy secondary to ascending aortic banding, subendocardial fibrosis has been reported.[26]

In the normal resting awake animal subendocardial blood flow is greater than subepicardial flow, reflecting greater systolic wall stress and oxygen requirements in the deeper myocardial layers.[27] This gradient of blood flow favoring the subendocardium is also maintained during treadmill exercise. In contrast, in the hypertrophied heart subendocardial blood flow undergoes a subnormal increase during exercise, resulting in a subendocardial/subepicardial blood flow ratio.[26,28-30] These observations illustrate the increased vulnerability of the hypertrophied heart to subendocardial hypoperfusion, which is particularly pronounced during periods of increased work, such as exercise.

Perfusion abnormalities in the hypertrophied heart could be caused by 1) an increase in minimum coronary vascular resistance, resulting from a decreased maximal cross-sectional area of the vascular bed per gram of myocardium. The latter can result from structural coronary alterations such as vascular rarefaction as the vascular bed fails to grow commensurately with the degree of myocardial hypertrophy, or a decrease in vascular lumen due to vascular medial hypertrophy resulting in lumenal encroachment; 2) an increase in extravascular intramyocardial forces that act to compress the vasculature and hence impede blood flow, or 3) alterations in vasomotor tone originating from either endothelial or vascular smooth muscle dysfunction.

Minimum coronary resistance

A decrease in maximal cross-sectional area of the coronary vascular bed results in an increased minimum resistance per gram of myocardium. Studies in canine models of pressure overload hypertrophy (Table 1) have generally found an increase in minimum coronary vascular resistance, derived from single measurements of pressure and flow during maximum coronary vasodilation.[31-39]

A more complete characterization of the resistive properties of the coronary vascular bed can be obtained by examining the pressure-flow relationship (Figure 3).[40-42] During maximal vasodilation the pressure-flow relationship is linear throughout most of its pressure range, but often with convexity toward the flow axis at low perfusion pressures.

Table 1. Reports of Minimum Coronary Vascular Resistance Computed From Single Coronary Pressure and Blood Flow Measurements in Canine Models of Left Ventricular Pressure-Overload Hypertrophy.

| Investigators | Hypertrophy stimulus | | | LVW/BW (g/kg) | CP (mm/Hg) | | maximum CBF (ml/min per gram) | | minimum CVR [mmHg/(ml/min per gram)] | |
	Type	Onset	Duration		Normal	LVH	Normal	LVH	Normal	LVH
Aortic stenosis										
Holtz et al[31]	SVAS	Puppy	12 Months	8.5	73	66	3.6	2.0	16	26*
O'Keefe et al[32]	SVAS	Adult	6 weeks	5.1	...	...	4.2	3.1	20	33*
Bache et al[33]	SVAS	Puppy	10-14 Months	8.3	89	125	6.1	5.4	15	23*
Bache et al[34]	SVAS	Puppy	10-14 Months	6.9	84	106	5.6	5.7	17	21*
Alyono et al[35]	SVAS	Adult	2 Months	6.6	84	126	5.6	5.9	17	22*
	VAS	Puppy	10-14 Months	7.1	87	78	6.7	3.3*	13	24*
Renovascular hypertension										
Mueller et al[36]	1K1C	Adult	6-7 Weeks	6.1	72	108	5.6	4.9	15	26*
Marcus et al[37]	2K1C	Adult	6 Weeks	5.1	77	81	5.4	3.5	16	24*
	2K1C	Adult	6 Months	5.1	77	88	5.4	3.7	16	25*
Tomanek et al[38]	1K1C	Adult	6 Weeks	5.8	52	83	3.7	3.9	15	25*
Tomanek et al[39]	1K1C	Adult	7 Months	6.7	78	95	5.9	5.8	14	17

LVW/BW, left ventricular to body weight ratio; CP, coronary pressure; LVH, left ventricular hypertrophy; CBF, coronary blood flow; CVR, coronary vascular resistance (calculated as CP/CBF, except in the study by O'Keefe et al,[32] in which CVR was calculated as CP minus left ventricular end-diastolic pressure divided by CBF); SVAS, supravalvular aortic stenosis; VAS, valvular aortic stenosis; 1K1C, one-kidney, one-clip model; 2K1C two-kidney, one-clip model.

O'Keefe et al[32] studied anesthetized dogs during coronary vasodilation with adenosine or carbochromene. All other studies were performed in vivo in awake or sedated dogs while adenosine or dipyridamole (Holtz et al[31]) was used to induce maximal vasodilation. In the study of Holtz et al,[31] diastolic aortic pressure was used as coronary perfusion pressure, while flow and resistance data for the subendocardium were reported. All other studies presented mean CPs and mean transmural CBF and CVR data. Note that LVW/BW ratio's are 4.0-5.0 g/kg in normal dogs. *p<0.05 vs. normal dogs. (Modified from Duncker et al.[42])

CORONARY PRESSURE-FLOW RELATIONSHIP

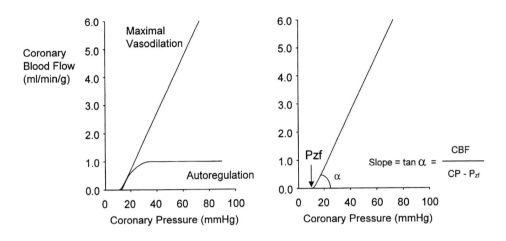

Figure 3. Coronary pressure-flow relation. In the left panel is shown the coronary pressure-flow relation under conditions of intact vasomotor tone (i.e. with intact autoregulation) and during maximal coronary vasodilation (e.g. with adenosine). Note that during maximal vasodilation, coronary blood flow is a linear function of coronary pressure (CP). In the right panel is shown how the pressure-flow relation can be described by the slope of the relation (tan α which reflects the maximum conductance, or the inverse of minimum coronary resistance) and the coronary pressure at which flow stops (pressure at zero flow, Pzf). Decreases in maximum blood flow can be due to an increase in minimum resistance and / or an increase in Pzf.

The slope of the pressure-flow relationship (change in flow/change in pressure) represents maximum conductance (which is the inverse of minimum resistance), while perfusion pressure at zero flow (Pzf) reflects the back pressure opposing coronary blood flow, and which is usually 5-10 mmHg higher than right atrial pressure. Coronary pressure-flow relationships differentiate between changes in minimum resistance and alterations in the back pressure which opposes flow, allowing a more comprehensive understanding of the mechanisms responsible for abnormal perfusion in the hypertrophied heart. Thus, structural vascular changes which result in a decrease in the maximal cross-sectional area of the vasculature (vascular rarefaction or decreased resistance vessel lumen/wall thickness ratio) would result in a decreased slope, whereas an increase in extravascular compressive forces would result in a higher Pzf.[40-42]

Several investigators have examined coronary pressure-flow relationships during maximal vasodilation with adenosine in canine models of pressure overload hypertrophy produced by aortic banding or renovascular hypertrension (Table 2).[42-46] These studies (with the exception of one[45]) demonstrated a decreased slope, indicating that maximum conductance is decreased, i.e. that minimum resistance is increased (Figure 4).[42-44, 46]

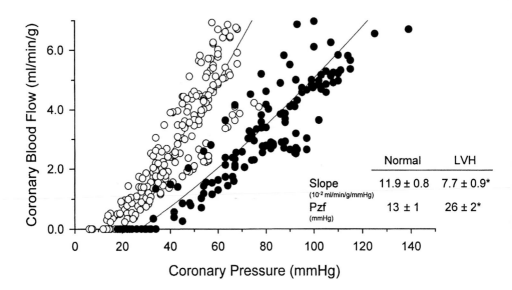

Figure 4. Pressure-flow data points from 11 normal dogs (O) and 7 dogs with left ventricular (LV) hypertrophy (●) under resting conditions. Data were obtained during maximal coronary vasodilation with adenosine. The slope and P_{zf} presented in the inserted table represent the averaged values of the individual dogs. Data are from Duncker et al.[44]

Vascular rarefaction

An increase in minimum resistance could result from vascular rarefaction as the coronary vessels fail to grow in proportion to the degree of hypertrophy. This is supported by the inverse relation between the slope of the pressure-flow relationship and the left ventricular to body weight ratio (Figure 5). However, studies of hypertrophied myocardium of renovascular hypertensive rats[47] and dogs,[38] as well as swine subjected to ascending aortic banding,[48] failed to demonstrate decreases in the densities of arterioles, in which the major part of resistance resides. However, the degree of hypertrophy in these studies was moderate, with increments of left ventricle to body weight ratios of 45%-50%.[38,47,48]

Table 2. Coronary Pressure-Flow Relations in Canine Models of Left Ventricular Pressure-Overload Hypertrophy.

Investigators	Hypertrophy stimulus			Hypertrophy LVW/BW (g/kg)	Experimental conditions	Slope [mmHg/(ml/min per gram)]		P_{zf} (mmHg)	
	Type	Onset	Duration			Normal	LVH	Normal	LVH
Aortic stenosis									
Scheel et al[43]	SVAS	Adult	4 Weeks	6.2	Diastolic measurements, empty beating hearts	12.4	7.7*	17	19*
Duncker et al[42]	SVAS	Puppy	10-14 Months	8.7	Transmural measurements, in vivo hearts, open-chest dogs	9.3	5.8*	12	24*
Duncker et al[44]	SVAS	Puppy	10-14 Months	7.7	Transmural measurements, in vivo hearts, awake dogs	11.9	7.7*	13	26*
Renovascular hypertension									
Harrison et al[45]	1K1C	Adult	6-8 Weeks	5.6	Transmural measurements, empty beating hearts	6.5	6.2	17.7	18.2
Jeremy et al[46]	1K1C	Adult	6-12 Weeks	5.5	Diastolic measurements, extracorporeal perfusion	13.5	8.5*	17.8	15.2

LVW/BW, left ventricular to body weight ratio; P_{zf}, coronary pressure at zero flow; SVAS, supravalvular aortic stenosis; 1K1C, one-kidney, one-clip model. In normal dogs LVW/BW ratio's are 4.0-5.0 g/kg. *p<0.05 vs. normal dogs. (Modified from Duncker et al.[42])

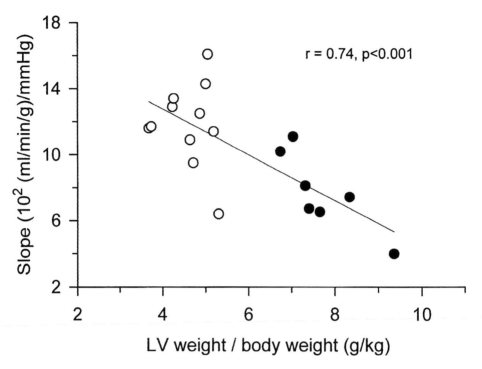

Figure 5. Correlation between LV weight (LVW)-to-body weight ratio and slope of pressure-flow relationship for individual data of normal animals (O) and animals with LV hypertrophy (●). Data were obtained during maximal coronary vasodilation with adenosine. Data are from Duncker et al.[44]

Alternatively, as the coronary vasculature increases its length in the face of the increase in left ventricular mass, vascular resistance increases in a linear fashion. It is therefore possible that minimum resistance could increase even without a decrease in coronary arteriolar density.

Vascular medial hypertrophy

Perfusion abnormalities could also occur from chronic exposure of the coronary vasculature to high perfusion pressures, independent of the degree of myocardial hypertrophy.[49,50] Indeed, vascular medial hypertrophy has been described in coronary arterioles of hypertensive rats.[47,51-53] That this may be a species specific phenomenon is suggested by the observation that in large animal models such as swine subjected to aortic banding[48] and renovascular hypertensive dogs[38,39] normal wall/lumen ratios are generally reported. Bishop et al[54] banded the ascending aorta of young dogs at 8 weeks of age which resulted in a 68% increase in relative left ventricular mass 10-14 months later. Although small arteries (outer diameter >100 μm) showed an increased wall/lumen ratio, arterioles (outer diameter <100 μm) showed a normal wall/lumen ratios. Furthermore, an increase in wall/lumen ratio does not necessarily imply narrowing of the lumen, as outward remodeling of the vessel may accompany the medial hypertrophy thereby leaving the lumenal diameter constant.[38,55] In pressure-overload hypertrophied canine left ventricles, the degree of hypertropy but not hypertensive vascular changes appear to be responsible for the increased minimum resistance. This is suggested by the inverse relation between the slope of the pressure-flow relationship and the degree of hypertrophy on the one hand, and the lack of correlation between the slope and coronary artery pressure on the other, suggesting that hypertrophy and not exposure to high intravascular pressure within the coronary bed was responsible for the decreased increased minimum resistance.[44] This conclusion is also supported by the study of Alyono et al.[35] who observed that perfusion abnormalities occurred in dogs with left ventricular hypertrophy secondary to valvular aortic stenosis in which coronary pressures are not increased.

Increased vasomotor tone

Alterations in vasomotor tone may also contribute to perfusion abnormalities in the compensated hypertrophied left ventricle. Thus, during exercise, α_1-adrenergic coronary vasoconstriction is greater in dogs with pressure-overload left ventricular hypertrophy than in normal dogs,[30,56] supporting a role for exaggerated increments in adrenergic vasomotor tone as a cause for subendocardial hypoperfusion during exercise (Figure 6).[30]

Besides an increased vasoconstrictor influence, myocardial hypoperfusion could also result from loss of vasodilator capacity. Thus, impairment of endothelium-dependent vasodilation of coronary resistance vessels has been observed in patients with hypertension[57-59] and in patients with left ventricular hypertrophy,[59] resulting from reduced expression of endothelial constitutive nitric oxide synthase.[60]

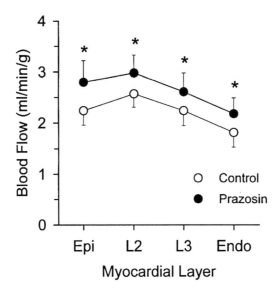

Figure 6. Myocardial blood flow in four layers across the left ventricular anterior wall of seven exercising dogs with left ventricular hypertrophy, from outer (epi) to inner (endo) layer. Myocardial blood flow is shown during control exercise (open circles) and during exercise in the presence of the α_1-adrenoceptor antagonist prazosin (10 µg/kg intracoronary) (closed circles). Prazosin produced similar increases in blood flow to all myocardial layers, indicating that α_1-adrenergic tone limits blood flow to a similar extent in all myocardial layers. Data are from Duncker et al.[30]

Extravascular compressive forces

An increase in extravascular intramyocardial forces that act to compress the vasculature could contribute to the increased impediment of coronary blood flow in the compensated hypertrophied left ventricle. A number of studies investigated the pressure-flow relation and reported an increased Pzf (Table 2). Scheel et al.[43] and Jeremy et al.[46] reported late diastolic coronary pressure-flow measurements, which are susceptible to capacitance effects.[41] Thus, flowmeter measurements on a proximal coronary artery do not take into account capacitive discharge (unloading) of blood from the distal vasculature as pressure falls during diastole, thereby underestimating the diastolic blood flow in the coronary microcirculation. Furthermore, capacitance effects are likely to be greater in hypertrophied than in normal hearts, due to greater amplitude of the systolic-diastolic pressure oscillations. Capacitance effects were minimized in the study of Scheel et al.[43] who performed measurements in empty left ventricles vented to atmospheric pressure. Full cycle

diastolic pressure.[66] Thus, increased compressive forces in the hyperthropied left ventricle during excercise result from both hemodynamic conditions and altered diastolic duration, due to a slower of contraction and relaxation.

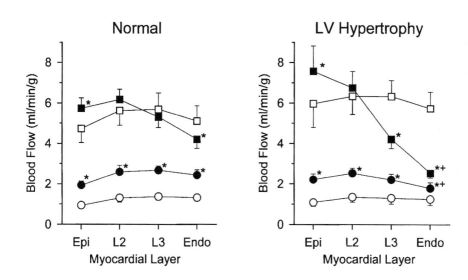

Figure 8. Myocardial blood flow in 4 layers across the left ventrcular (LV) anterior wall of 9 normal dogs (A) and 6 dogs with LV hypertrophy (LVH; B) from outer [subEpicardial (Epi)] to inner [subendocardial (Endo)] layer. Myocardial blood flow data are shown at rest (open symbols) and during exercise (solid symbols), both in absence (circles) and presence (squares) of intracoronary adenosine (50-100 µg kg^{-1} min^{-1}). L2, layer 2, outer midmyocardium; L3, layer 3, inner midmyocardium. *P < 0.05, exercise vs. rest; †P < 0.05, LVH vs normal. Data are from Duncker et al.[66]

How do perfusion abnormalities lead to sustained systolic dysfunction?

In the normal heart brief periods of ischemia that are too brief to cause myocardial necrosis, result in post-ischemic contractile dysfunction (myocardial stunning) that can persist for hours or days. Exercise in the presence of a coronary artery stenosis can also produce myocardial stunning.[67] Furthermore, exercise-induced stunning is cumulative, i.e. repeated periods of exercise can result in progressively more severe dysfunction.[68] Repetitive periods of stress-induced ischemia may thus lead to progressive loss of contractile function and ATP in the subendocardium of the hypertrophied left ventricle. This is further excacerbated by the exaggerated increments in oxygen requirements of the hypertrophied myocardium during exercise.[29] In support of this possible chain of events, Hittinger et al.[26] described that with the development of contractile dysfunction a further loss of subendocardial vasodilator reserve occurred possibly leading to even greater susceptibility to subendocardial ischemia, which can eventually lead to irreversibly damaged myocardium, evidenced by subendocardial fibrosis in their study. But even when necrosis does not occur, repetitive stunning could lead to a state of prolonged downregulation of function called hibernation.[69] Hibernation is characterized by increased interstitial collagen content and an increased glucose uptake,[70] features that are also found in severely hypertrophied left ventricles.[20,71] Once the myocardium enters a state of hibernation, systolic contractile performance starts to deteriorate leading to an increased systolic wall stress thereby eliciting further hypertrophic remodeling. In this way, subendocardial perfusion abnormalities could eventually lead to a sustained systolic dysfunction in the hypertrophied left ventricle.

Conclusions

In the compensated pressure-overload hypertrophied left ventricle, global systolic pump function appears normal for a prolonged period of time although contraction is slower which may serve to produce greater economy of contraction. Abnormalities of diastolic function which occur much earlier in the process of hypertrophic remodeling of the left ventricle, are characterized by an increased diastolic left ventricular stiffness. The impairment of diastolic function could act to impede filling of the left ventricle during periods of increased work load. In addition, perfusion abnormalities can be excacerbated by increasing the extravascular compressive forces in the hypertrophied ventricle, particularly during periods of increased work when heart rate increments reduce diastolic perfusion time. Perfusion abnormalities arise further from increased minimum resistance and increased coronary vasomotor tone. The consequent recurrent periods of subendocardial ischemia may lead to progressive dysfunction of the hypertrophied left ventricle.

References

1. Kannel WB, Cobb J. Left ventricular hypertrophy and mortality--results from the Framingham Study. Cardiology 1992;81:291-8.
2. Fujii AM, Vatner SF, Serur J, Als A, Mirsky I. Mechanical and inotropic reserve in conscious dogs with left ventricular hypertrophy. Am J Physiol 1986;251:H815-23.
3. Spann JF Jr, Buccino RA, Sonnenblick EH, Braunwald E. Contractile state of cardiac muscle obtained from cats with experimentally produced ventricular hypertrophy and heart failure. Circ Res 1967;21:341-54.
4. Burger SB, Strauer BE. Left ventricular hypertrophy in chronic pressure load due to spontaneous essential hypertension. II. Contractility of the isolated left ventricular myocardium and left ventricular stiffness. In: Strauer BE, editor. The heart in hypertension. Berlin: Springer: 1981. p. 37-52.
5. Harding S, Poole-Wilson P. Myocyte contractile dysfunction in cardiac hypertrophy. In: Sheridan DJ, editor. Left ventricular hypertrophy. Edinburgh: Churchill Livingston; 1998. p. 85-91.
6. Siri FM, Krueger J, Nordin C, Ming Z, Aronson RS. Depressed intracellular calcium transients and contraction in myocytes from hypertrophied and failing guinea pig hearts. Am J Physiol 1991;261:H514-30.
7. Weinberg EO, Schoen FJ, George D, et al. Angiotensin-converting enzyme inhibition prolongs survival and modifies the transition to heart failure in rats with pressure overload hypertrophy due to ascending aortic stenosis. Circulation 1994;90:1410-22.
8. Gwathmey JK, Morgan JP. Altered calcium handling in experimental pressure-overload hypertrophy in the ferret. Circ Res 1985;57:836-43.
9. Alpert NR, Mulieri LA, Hasenfuss G. Myocardial chemo-mechanical energy transduction. In: Fozzard HA, et al., editors. The heart and cardiovascular system. New York: Raven Press 1992. p. 111-28.
10. Swynghedauw B. Moalic JM, Celcayre C. The origins of cardiac hypertrophy. In: Swynghedauw B, ed. Research in cardiac hypertrophy and failure. London: INSERM/John Libbey Eurotext, 1990:23-50.
11. Mondry A, Swynghedauw B. Biological adaptation of the myocardium to chronic mechanical overload. Molecular determinants of the autonomic nervous system. Eur Heart J 1995;16:64-73.
12. Ventura-Clapier R, Mekhfi H, Oliviero P, Swynghedauw B. Pressure overload changes cardiac skinned-fiber mechanics in rats, not in guinea pigs. Am J Physiol 1988;254:H517-24.
13. Klug D, Robert V, Swynghedauw B. Role of mechanical and hormonal factors in cardiac remodeling and the biologic limits of myocardial adaptation. Am J Cardiol 1993;71:46A-54A.
14. Schaub MC, Hefti MA, Zuellig RA, Morano I. Modulation of contractility in human cardiac hypertrophy by myosin essential light chain isoforms. Cardiovasc Res 1998;37:381-404.
15. Callens-el Amrani F, Mayoux E, et al. Normal responsiveness to external Ca and to Ca-channel modifying agents in hypertrophied rat heart. Am J Physiol 1990;258:H1727-34.
16. Naudin V, Oliviero P, Rannou F, Sainte Beuve C, Charlemagne D. The density of ryanodine receptors decreases with pressure overload-induced rat cardiac hypertrophy. FEBS Lett 1991;285:135-8.
17. Nuss HB, Houser SR. Voltage dependence of contraction and calcium current in severely hypertrophied feline ventricular myocytes. J Mol Cell Cardiol 1991;23:717-26.
18. Gomez AM, Valdivia HH, Cheng H, et al. Defective excitation-contraction coupling in experimental cardiac hypertrophy and heart failure. Science 1997;276:800-6.
19. Gaasch WH, Levine HJ, Quinones MA, Alexander JK. Left ventricular compliance: mechanisms and clinical implications. Am J Cardiol 1976;38:645-53.
20. Weber KT, Janicki JS, Shroff SG, Pick R, Chen RM, Bashey RI. Collagen remodeling of the pressure-overloaded, hypertrophied nonhuman primate myocardium. Circ Res 1988;62:757-65.
21. Nagai R, Zarain-Herzberg A, Brandl CJ, et al. Regulation of myocardial Ca^{2+}-ATPase and phospholamban mRNA expression in response to pressure overload and thyroid hormone. Proc Natl Acad Sci U S A 1989;86:2966-2970.
22. De la Bastie D, Levitsky D, Rappaport L, Mercadier JJ, Marotte F, Wisnewsky C, Brovkovich V, Schwartz K, Lompre AM. Function of the sarcoplasmic reticulum and expression of its Ca2(+)-ATPase gene in pressure overload-induced cardiac hypertrophy in the rat. Circ Res 1990;66:554-64.
23. Goodwin JR. Hypertrophic diseases of the myocardium. Prog Cardiovasc Dis 1973;16:199-238.
24. Harris CN, Aronow WS, Parker DP, Kaplan MA. Treadmill stress tests in left ventricular hypertrophy. Chest 1973;63:353-7.
25. Mollar JH, Nakeb A, Edwards JE. Infarction of the papillary muscle and mitral insufficiency associated with congenital aortic stenosis. Circulation 1966;34:87-91.
26. Hittinger L, Shannon RP, Bishop SP, Gelpi RJ, Vatner SF. Subendomyocardial exhaustion of blood flow reserve and increased fibrosis in conscious dogs with heart failure. Circ Res 1989;65:971-80.
27. Laughlin MH, Korthuis RJ, Duncker DJ, Bache RJ. Regulation of blood flow to cardiac and skeletal muscle

during exercise. In: Rowell LB, Shepherd JT, editors. Exercise: regulation and integration of multiple systems. New York: Oxford University Press; 1996. p. 705-69.

28.   Bache RJ, Dai XZ, Alyono D, Vrobel TR, Homans DC. Myocardial blood flow during exercise in dogs with left ventricular hypertrophy produced by aortic banding and perinephritic hypertension. Circulation 1987;76:835-42.

29.   Bache RJ, Dai X.Z. Myocardial oxygen consumption during exercise in the presence of left ventricular hypertrophy secondary to supravalvular aortic stenosis. J Am Coll Cardiol 1990;15:1157-64.

30.   Duncker DJ, Zhang J, Crampton M, Bache RJ. α_1-adrenergic activity restricts subendocardial blood flow in the hypertrophied left ventricle of exercising dogs. Basic Res Cardiol 1995;90;73-83.

31.   Holtz J, Restorff W, Bard P, Bassenge E. Transmural distribution of myocardial blood flow and of coronary reserve in canine left ventricular hypertrophy. Basic Res Cardiol 1977;72:286-92.

32.   O'Keefe, DO, Hoffman JIE, Cheitlin, O'Neill MJ, Allard JR, Shapkin E. Coronary blood flow in experimental canine left ventricular hypertrophy. Circ Res 1978;43: 43-51.

33.   Bache RJ, Vrobel TR, Arentzen CE, Ring WS. Effect of maximal coronary vasodilation on transmural myocardial perfusion during tachycardia in dogs with left ventricular hypertrophy. Circ Res 1981;49:742-50.

34.   Bache RJ, Alyono D, Sublett E, Dai XZ. Myocardial blood flow in left ventricular hypertrophy developing in young and adult dogs. Am J Physiol 1986;251:H949-56.

35.   Alyono D, Anderson RW, Parrish DG, Dai XZ, Bache RJ. Alterations of myocardial blood flow associated with experimental canine left ventricular hypertrophy secondary to valvular aortic stenosis. Circ Res 1986;58:47-57.

36.   Mueller TM, Marcus ML, Kerber RE, Young JA, Barnes RW, Abboud FM. Effect of renal hypertension and left ventricular hypertrophy on the coronary circulation. Circ Res 1978;42:543-9.

37.   Marcus ML, Mueller TM, Eastham CL. Effects of short- and long-term left ventricular hypertrophy on coronary circulation. Am J Physiol 1981;241:H358-62.

38.   Tomanek RJ, Palmer PJ, Peiffer GL, Schreiber KL, Eastham CL, Marcus ML. Morphometry of canine coronary arteries arterioles and capillaries during hypertension and left ventricular hypertrophy. Circ Res 1986;58: 38-46.

39.   Tomanek RJ, Schalk KA, Marcus ML, Harrison DG. Coronary angiogenesis during long-term hypertension and left ventricular hypertrophy in dogs. Circ Res 1989;65:352-9.

40.   Klocke FJ. Measurements of coronary flow reserve: defining pathophysiology versus making decisions about patient care. Circulation 1987;76:1183-9.

41.   Hoffman JIE, Spaan JAE. Pressure-flow relations in coronary circulation. Physiol Rev 1990;70:331-90.

42.   Duncker DJ, Zhang J, Bache RJ. Pressure-flow relationship in left ventricular hypertrophy. Importance of changes in backpressure versus changes in minimum resistance. Circ Res 1993;72:579-587.

43.   Scheel KW, Eisenstein BL, Ingram LA. Coronary, collateral, and perfusion territory responses to aortic banding. Am J Physiol 1984;246:H768-75.

44.   Duncker DJ, Zhang J, Pavek T, Crampton MJ, Bache RJ. Effect of exercise on coronary pressure-flow relationship in hypertrophied left ventricle. Am J Physiol 1995;269:H271-81.

45.   Harrison DG, Barnes DH, Hiratzka LF, Eastham CL, Kerber RE, Marcus ML. The effect of cardiac hypertrophy on the coronary circulation. Circulation 1985;71:1135-45.

46.   Jeremy RW, Fletcher PJ, Thompson J. Coronary pressure-flow relations in hypertensive left ventricular hypertrophy. Circ Res 1989;65: 224-36.

47.   Rakusan K, Cheng M, Wicker P, Healy B. Morphometry of coronary arterioles in normal and hypertorphic rat heart. In: Tsuchiya M, et al., editor. Microcirculation: an update, volume 2. Amsterdam: Excerpta Medica; 1987. p. 185-6.

48.   Breisch EA, White FC, Nimmo LE, Bloor CM. Cardiac vasculature and flow during pressure-overload hypertrophy. Am J Physiol 1986;251:H1031-7.

49.   Strauer BE. Left ventricular dynamics, energetics and coronary hemodynamics in hypertrophied heart disease. Eur Heart J 1983;4:137-42.

50.   Folkow B, Hallback M, Lundgren Y, Weiss L. Structurally based increase of flow resistance in spontaneously hypertensive rats. Acta Physiol Scand 1970;79:373-9.

51.   Tomanek RJ, Wrangler RD, Bauer CA. Prevention of coronary vasodilator reserve decrements in spontaneously hypertensive rats. Hypertension 1985;7:533-40.

52.   Anderson PG, Bishop SP, Digerness SB. Cardiac and vascular pathology of hydralazine treated DOCA salt rats. J Mol Cell Cardiol 1988;20:755-67.

53.   Brilla CG, Hanicki JS, Weber KT. Impaired diastolic function and coronary reserve in genetic hypertension. Role of interstitial fibrosis and medial thickening of intramyocardial coronary arteries. Circ Res 1991;69:107-15.

54.   Bishop SP, Powell PC, Hasebe N, Shen YT Hittinger L, Vatner SF. Coronary vascular morphology and

reduced coronary reserve in dogs with chronic pressure overload cardiac hypertrophy [abstract]. Circulation 1993;88:I545.

55.   Vlodaver Z, Neufeld HN. The coronary arteries in coarctation of the aorta. Circulation 1968;37:449-54.

56.   Bache RJ, Homans DC, Dai XZ. Adrenergic vasoconstriction limits coronary blood flow during exercise in hypertrophied left ventricle. Am J Physiol 1991;260:H1489-94.

57.   Treasure CB, Manoukian SV, Klein JL, Vita JA, Nabel EG, Renwick GH, Selwyn AP, Alexander RW, Ganz P. Epicardial coronary artery responses to acetylcholine are impaired in hypertensive patients. Circ Res 1992;71:776-81.

58.   Egashira K, Suzuki S, Hirooka Y, Kai H, Sugimachi M, Imaizumi T, Takeshita A. Impaired endothelium-dependent vasodilation of large epicardial and resistance coronary arteries in patients with essential hypertension. Different responses to acetylcholine and substance P. Hypertension 1995;25:201-6.

59.   Treasure CB, Klein JL, Vita JA, Manoukian SV, Renwick GH, Selwyn AP, Ganz P, Alexander RW. Hypertension and left ventricular hypertrophy are associated with impaired endothelium-mediated relaxation in human coronary resistance vessels. Circulation 1993;87:86-93.

60.   Crabos M, Coste P, Paccalin M, Tariosse L, Daret D, Besse P, Bonoron-Adele S. Reduced basal NO-mediated dilation and decreased endothelial NO-synthase expression in coronary vessels of spontaneously hypertensive rats. J Mol Cell Cardiol 1997;29:55-65.

61.   Ellis AK, Klocke FJ. Effects of preload on the transmural distribution of perfusion and pressure-flow relationships in the canine coronary vascular bed. Circ Res 1979;46:68-77.

62.   Uhlig PN, Baer RW, Vlahakes GJ, Hanley FL, Messina LM, Hoffman JIE. Arterial and venous coronary pressure-flow relations in anesthetized dogs. Evidence for a vascular waterfall in epicardial coronary veins. Circ Res 1984;55:238-48.

63.   Satoh S, Watanabe J, Keitoku M, Itoh N, Maruyama Y, Takishima T. Influences of pressure surrounding the heart and intracardiac pressure on the diastolic coronary pressure-flow relation in excised canine heart. Circ Res 1988;63:788-97.

64.   Watanabe J, Maruyama Y, Satoh S, Keitoku M, Takishima T. Effects of the pericardium on the diastolic left coronary pressure-flow relationship in the isolated dog heart. Circulation 1987;75:670-5.

65.   Archie JP Jr. Transmural distribution of intrinsic and transmitted left ventricular diastolic intramyocardial pressure in dogs. Cardiovasc Res 1978;12:255-62.

66.   Duncker DJ, Ishibashi Y, Bache RJ. Effect of treadmill exercise on transmural distribution of blood flow in hypertrophied left ventricle. Am J Physiol 1998;275:H1274-82.

67.   Homans DC, Sublett E, Dai XZ, Bache RJ. Persistence of regional left ventricular dysfunction after exercise-induced myocardial ischemia. J Clin Invest 1986;77:66-73.

68.   Homans DC, Laxson DD, Sublett E, Lindstrom P, Bache RJ. Cumulative deterioration of myocardial function after repeated episodes of exercise-induced ischemia. Am J Physiol 1989;256:H1462-71.

69.   Shen YT, Vatner SF. Mechanism of impaired myocardial function during progressive coronary stenosis in conscious pigs. Hibernation versus stunning? Circ Res 1995;76:479-88.

70.   Fallavollita JA, Perry BJ, Canty JM Jr. 18F-2-deoxyglucose deposition and regional flow in pigs with chronically dysfunctional myocardium. Evidence for transmural variations in chronic hibernating myocardium. Circulation 1997;95:1900-9.

71.   Zhang J, Duncker DJ, Ya X, et al. Effect of left ventricular hypertrophy secondary to chronic pressure overload on transmural myocardial 2-deoxyglucose uptake. A 31P NMR spectroscopic study. Circulation 1995;92:1274-83.

4. ASSESSMENT OF LEFT VENTRICULAR HYPERTROPHY: A COMPARISON OF ELECTROCARDIOGRAPHY, ECHOCARDIOGRAPHY AND MAGNETIC RESONANCE IMAGING

A.J. BREES, B.M. PLUIM, H.W. VLIEGEN, A. DE ROOS, H.J. LAMB, E.E. VAN DER WALL

Summary

Left ventricular hypertrophy (LVH) can be morphologically described as an increase in muscle mass of the left ventricle (LV).[1] Three common approaches used to determine LVH are the electrocardiogram (ECG), the echocardiogram and magnetic resonance imaging (MRI). There are differences in the results obtained by all three techniques as illustrated by the fact that LVH prevalence in the general population increases with age by approximately 1 to 10% if determined using ECG,[2] and from 5 to almost 50% according to echocardiographic data.[3] It has also been demonstrated that echocardiography is considerably less precise in measuring LV mass than MRI, and is therefore considerably less reliable. This suggests that echocardiography would be better for measuring changes in LV mass in groups of patients, but is limited in its use for clinical evaluation of the individual patient.

The ECG is widely used in primary screening procedures since it requires relatively little expertise, is cheap and the results are easy to interpret. MRI provides highly accurate LV mass easurements and permits tissue imaging but its use is limited by restricted availability, fixed facilities and claustrophobia-inducing effects.

Introduction

In the last 10 years, many different researchers using many different populations have

E. E. van der Wall et al.(eds.), Left Ventricular Hypertrophy, 43-53.
© 1999 *Kluwer Academic Publishers. Printed in the Netherlands.*

elucidated a strong and consistent relationship identified between increased LV mass at baseline examination and a heightened risk of subsequent cardiovascular events. This relationship has been demonstrated for hypertensive patients,[4] normal healthy individuals,[5] and groups of patients with documented coronary heart disease.[6] Results from additional studies have shown that changes with time in LV mass,[7] or electrophysiological indices thereof,[8] are related directly to subsequent risk complications. These observations have emphasized the importance of an accurate method of establishing LV mass. It is the purpose of this chapter to present and compare the three most commonly used techniques (i.e. electrocardiography, echocardiography, magnetic resonance imaging) for detection of LVH, and to evaluate their relative strengths and weaknesses.

Electrocardiography

There are several criteria for electrocardiographic left ventricular hypertrophy (ECG-LVH) which are usually related to the height and width of the QRS complex and abnormalities in the ST-T segment.[9] Hypertrophied myocardial cells, a thicker wall or increased wall stress are accepted as providing taller and wider QRS complexes, and smaller T-wave peaks.

ST-T abnormalities indicate repolarization problems and may appear in hemodynamic overload, myocardial ischemia and myocardial damage as well as in LVH.[10] Classic indications of ECG-LVH are ST-T segment depression in leads V4-V6, commonly referred to as "LV strain". Specifically, ECG-LVH is usually identified by fulfilling one of three potential criteria:

1. The Sokolow-Lyon criteria: SV1 + RV5 or RV6 ≥35mV,

2) Romhilt-Estes score: ≥5 (points are given for different ECG abnormalities. In particular attention is paid to high voltage, the height of the P-wave-top in V1, repolarization and the use of digitalis),

3) Cornell-voltage criteria (RaVL + SV3 > 28mV for men and > 20mV for women).

The sensitivity of ECG for hypertrophy according to literature varies from 21-54%, with the sensitivity increasing as the degree of hypertrophy increases, although this is not apparent in all ECG-LVH criteria.[11,12,13] According to Devereux et al.,[12] the sensitivity of ECG, when using the Cornell-voltage criteria for ECG-LVH, increased from 27% for small LVH [2-3 standard deviations (SD) above the mean to 57% for significant LVH (>4SD above the mean)], at a specificity of 97%, indicating a low risk of false positive readings. These data are fairly consistent with other studies.[11,13]

ECG-LVH has a greater capacity for predicting an increase risk of cardiovascular disease than echocardiography–assessed LVH, especially if there are repolarization disturbances evident.[10,14,15,16] The Framingham study, indicated that one-third of the men and a quarter of the women with LVH, with evident repolarization disturbances on the ECG, died within 5 years of the diagnosis.[10,14]

Echocardiography

Echocardiographic measurements of LVH is used only in second line investigations at this point in time and can only be performed by an experienced investigator. The LV mass (in grams) is estimated with the help of the thickness of usually the septum and posterior wall, the internal diameter and geometrical models. Measurement of LV mass by two-dimensional (2D) echocardiography depends on careful experimental calibration of the echocardiographic instrument using either a standard phantom or actual heart slices, and appropriate geometric algorithm, and short axis images to determine myocardial cross-sectional area.[17] Upper limits of normal LV mass have been described to be slightly lower (102 g/m^2 in males and 88 g/m^2 in females) than when determined by M-mode techniques (150 g/m^2 in males, 120 g/m^2 in females).[18] The 2D technique may have limited accuracy in mass determination if ventricular shape is deformed or the architecture is irregular, as it may be in various disease states.[19] The same authors contended that it is possible to obtain LV mass estimates with a high degree of accuracy from randomly oriented views without practical restriction on transducer motion or major geometric assumptions.

Using three of the standard M-Mode formulae [(American Society of Echocardiography,[20] Penn convention (based on work by Devereux and Reichek[21]), and Teicholz,[22]], LV mass in 24 hypertensive subjects have been demonstrated to vary considerably (319 ± 21 g, 273 ± 19 g and 191 ± 11 g respectively).[23] The cube formula (D^3), which is the most widely used formula to assess LV mass using M-mode recording, has been cited as repeatedly and substantially overestimating LV mass.[24,25] According to Wikstrand,[25] the correct formula has been cited in previous studies,[26,27] but has since been overseen. Schillaci et al.[28] support the notion that geometrical assumptions lead to approximations and fallacies in assessing a three-dimensional (3D) structure like the left ventricle. However, they contend that with the application of a correction factor proposed by Devereux et al.[24] the average overestimation of LV mass would decrease significantly.[28] Missouris et al.[29] replied by stating that a constant correction factor is unjustified due to the variable geometry of the heart, particularly in hypertensive subjects, as recognized by Genau et al.[30] Schnellbaecher et al.[31] lent further support for the inherent unreliability of the standard echocardiographic methods for the measurement of LV mass.

Diagnosis of echocardiographic diagnosed LVH is related to body surface area (in m^2), Quetelet-index (in kg/m^2) or height (in m). The subsequent LV mass index provides a diagnosis related to the size of the subject.

The sensitivity of echocardiography is related to the degree of hypertrophy. Echocardiography of light hypertrophy (2-3 SD above the mean) demonstrated a sensitivity of 57%, whereas a sensitivity of 100% was demonstrated with extreme hypertrophy.[12] The specificity of echocardiography in determining LVH has been discovered to be high, resulting in a 3-16% chance of a false positive result.[12,] As well as providing information on LV mass, echocardiography can also provide information about wall motion and thickness abnormalities, valvular malfunctions, and systolic and diastolic performance.

Magnetic resonance imaging

Several validation studies have compared ventricular masses determined by ante-mortem MRI with angiographic LV mass of patients,[32] and by ex-vivo imaging of post-mortem human hearts.[33] These studies demonstrated correlation coefficients in the range of r=0.95-0.99, and standard error of the estimate (SEE) in the range of 1-13 g between MRI LV mass estimates and actual post-mortem ventricular weights. In-vivo validation studies have found close correlations between MRI-derived masses and actual heart weights; the SEE has been reported to be as low as 3 g,[34] comparing favorably with the best results obtained with the cine computed tomography technique. As noted above, MRI techniques have the theoretical advantage, when compared with ventriculography and conventional echocardiography, of permitting precise quantitation of masses and volumes of ventricles distorted by infarction.[35] Several studies have assessed the reproducibility of MRI LV mass measurements, with generally promising results.[34,36,37,38,39] Correlation coefficients for the intra-observer reproducibility have been in the range 0.96-0.99,[34] with variability of 3.5%,[37] and those for the inter-observer reproducibility in the range 0.97-0.99. The variability has been quantitated further with reported values for the inter-observer SEE of 5.4 g,[34] and 3.6% variability.[39]

One limitation of MRI has been the need for relatively long acquisition times using equipment that many patients find claustrophobic. There have been several studies attempting to alleviate this problem. Aurigemma et al.[40] reduced the imaging time by taking different MRI slices at sequential times through the cardiac cycle, and found close agreement of "single-phase" LV mass values with those obtained at enddiastole (r = 0.96, mean underestimation by 5 g).

Comparison of methods in the detection of LVH

Table 1 demonstrates that the specificity of ECG and echocardiography is high, and that there are relatively few false positive readings. The sensitivity of the ECG technique is noticeably lower than echocardiography and more false negative results are seen.Echocardiography, however, also reveals that in 7-15% of LVH cases a false negative result is demonstrated. In extreme cases of LVH, both echocardiography and ECG demonstrate improved diagnostic sensitivity, although some ECG criteria demonstrate limited diagnostic value.

Results obtained by MRI do appear to correlate closely to those of 2D-echocardiography. One study concerning children found an extremely close correlation (r = 0.98, SEE = 5.7 g) between LV mass estimates by MRI and by 2D-echocardiography.[41] Nonetheless, none of these studies were performed under the same difficult conditions as in grown-up patients.

Several studies have demonstrated that MRI appears to be a more reproducible tool of examination than M-mode echocardiography. [23,33,38,42] This was explained by the absence of geometrical assumptions for MRI, which is of particular importance in deformed ventricles. Two studies on athletes have shown different results with respect how the results obtained from the two techniques correlate. Turpeinen et al.[42] measured LV mass in seven endurance trained athletes and eight sedentary subjects using MRI and M-mode echocardiography. LV masses obtained by these two methods were only moderately correlated (r=0.47, p=0.05). Pluim et al.[43] however, demonstrated a correlation of 0.90 (mean difference 3.2 g, SD=21.9

Table 1. Sensitivity (%) and specificity (%) of electrocardiography (ECG) and echocardiography for detection of anatomic LVH using the post-mortem heart weight as reference standard.

First Author (no. of autopsies)	ECG		Echocardiography	
	Sensitivity	Specificity	Sensitivity	Specificity
Woythaler[13] (n=50)	54*	77	88	84
	54°	86		
	54#	86		
Devereux[12] (n=93)	22°	97	85	97
	34#	97		
	43&	97		
Reichek[11] (n=34)	21°	95	93	95
	50#	95		

*High voltage-ECG-LVH
° The Sokolow-Lyon criteria : SV1 + RV5 or RV6 ≥35mV.
Romhilt-Estes score: ≥5 points are give for different ECG abnormalities. In particular attention is paid to high voltage, the height of the P-wave-top in V1, repolarization and the use of digitalis
& Cornell-voltage criteria (RaVL + SV3 > 28mV for men and > 20mV for women)

g, p<0.0001) between M-mode LV mass calculations and MRI in 29 subjects. The possible difference in these results could be caused by the number of subjects, or the inter- and intra-observer reproducibility of the echocardiographic measurements.

In small studies comparing M-mode[44] (n=8) and 2D-echocardiographic methods (n=13),[45] the reproducibility of 2D methods has been shown to be moderately higher. However, in large population studies, the proportion of subjects whose LV masses can be determined by 2D methods have been found to be lower than that obtained with M-mode echocardiography.[46]

Several studies have compared 2D-echocardiography with MRI.[47,48,49] The main results of these studies indicated that in ventricles of normal shape, the cardiac dimension, mass and volume can be accurately assessed by both MRI and the echocardiography method for LV mass as proposed by the ASE.[20] This conclusion was supported by Pluim et al.[43] in athletes, demonstrating a correlation of 0.98 (p<0.0001, mean =3.4 g, SD 7.6 g).

Discussion

MRI has been shown to be a more reproducible tool than echocardiography in hypertensive patients,[23,49] and in normals,[33] while their predictive capacity is almost identical in athletes.[43] It appears that in pathologies with differing wall thicknesses and other deformations, the geometric models used to predict mass and volume of the left ventricle contribute to a loss in sensitivity. Echocardiography is more sensitive and approximately as specific as the ECG in measuring LVH. MRI has the disadvantage of being relatively limited in its availability, time consuming, expensive and claustrophobia inducing for the patient. Some authors will contend that MRI is more suitable for measuring LVH than echocardiography, as MRI is much more precise, accurate and reproducible as echocardiography. [50] By virtue of the greater accuracy of MRI, Bottini et al.[50] nicely showed that antihypertensive drug studies on reversibility of LV mass would require substantially less patients when using MRI instead of echocardiography. Furthermore, MRI is more suitable than echocardiography for assessment of LV mass and volumes in abnormally shaped ventricles. On the other hand there are authors who contend that (M-mode) echocardiography, in combination with 2D echocardiography (to exclude the possibility of left ventricular asymmetry), is a reliable and accurate method for studies of left ventricular morphology and function if used properly. Echocardiography is cheap, noninvasive and has a time resolution (real time) that is superior to any other method available.[25] Table 2 shows the strenghts and limitations of the various noninvasive methods for assessing LV mass.

Table 2. Strengths and limitations of noninvasive methods of LVM determination (taken in part from Devereux et al.[55]).

Technique	Advantages	Limitations
Electrocardiography	-Superior predictor of cardiovascular complications -Little expertise required -Widely available, suitable for large-scale use- -Relatively inexpensive	-Cannot provide morphological data -Relatively low sensitivity for prediction of LVH
M-Mode echocardiography	-Extensive anatomic validation -Known prognostic significance -Widely available, suitable for large scale use -Relatively inexpensive-	-Expertise-dependent -Errors in distorted ventricles
Two-dimensional echocardiography	-Some anatomic validation -Widely available	-Expertise-dependent -Time-consuming, limits large-scale use
Three-dimensional echocardiography	-High accuracy in limited anatomic validation -Anatomic validation	-Very time-consuming -Limited availability
Magnetic resonance Imaging	-High accuracy in limited anatomic validation -Tissue imaging possible	-Claustrophobia -Facilities expensive and fixed -3D measurements time-consuming -Limited availability

In clinical situations, where ECG is used as a diagnostic tool, the gold standard is often echocardiographic LVH. The sensitivity of ECG-LVH is 27-57% (lightly to highly hypertrophied left ventricles) and echocardiographic sensitivity lies between the 57% in lightly hypertrophied left ventricles, and 100% in highly hypertrophied left ventricles. As such the actual sensitivity of ECG measured LVH lies between the 17 and 73%, with a specificity of 86-99%.[9,11,51] Clearly ECG-LVH would be the third tool of choice for diagnosis. However, if ECG-LVH is detected, the risk for cardiovascular complications is 3-15 times as high as in subjects without ECG-LVH.[14] This relatively high risk factor is not evident in echocardiographic LVH.[47] Patients with both ECG-LVH and echocardiographic LVH are likely to experience arrhythmias 10 times as often as patients with only echocardiographic LVH.[52] The risk of sudden death in patients with ECG-LVH and repolarization disturbances increases by a factor 14 if ventricular ectopic tachycardia is evident as measured by Holter analysis.[53] ECG-LVH with associated repolarization disturbances has been indicated as the best predictor of cardiovascular complications.[54]

Conclusions

ECG evaluations of LVH have a practical value due to the nature of the availability, ease of use and relatively low cost. Echocardiography is useful in that it provides confirmation of LVH when used in combination with the ECG. In cases of extreme hypertrophy, undistorted ventricular geometry, and in the hands of experienced technicians, echocardiography is a reliable, simple, and noninvasive method to evaluate LVH. MRI is the most accurate and reliable method for evaluation of LVH, particularly in the advent of wall abnormalities. Unfortunately MRI is of limited availability, it is expensive and it requires considerable skill in its use. Future studies dealing with cost-effectiveness will determine the most appropriate technique for detection and evaluation of LVH.

References

1. Messerli FH, Ketelhut R. Left ventricular hypertrophy: a pressure-independent cardiovascular risk factor. J Cardiovasc Pharmacol 1993;22(Suppl)1:S7-13.
2. Kannel WB, Gordon T, Offutt D. Left ventricular hypertrophy by electrocardiography. Prevalence, incidence and mortality in the Framingham study. Ann Intern Med 1969;71:89-105
3. Levy D, Anderson KM, Savage DD, Kannel WB, Christiansen JC, Castelli WP. Echocardiographically detected left ventricular hypertrophy: prevalence and risk factors. The Framingham Heart Study. Ann Intern Med 1988;108:7-13.
4. Mensah GA, Pappas TW, Koren MJ, Ulin RJ, Laragh JH, Devereux RB. Comparison of classification of hypertension severity by blood pressure level and World Health Organisation criteria for prediction of concurrent cardiac abnormalities and subsequent complcations in essential hypertension. J Hypertens 1993;11:1433-44.
5. Levy D, Garrison RJ, Savage DD, Kannel WB, Castelli WP. Prognostic implications of echocardiographically determined left ventricular mass in the Framingham Heart Study. N Engl J Med 1990;322:1561-6.
6. Bolognese L, Dellavese P, Rossi L, Sarasso G, Bongo AS, Scianaro MC. Prognostic value of left ventricular mass in uncomplicated acute myocardial infarction and one-vessel coronary artery disease. Am J Cardiol 1994;73:1-5.
7. Muiesan ML, Salvetti M, Rizzoni D, Castellano M, Donato F, Agabiti-Rosei E. Association of change in left ventricular mass with prognosis during long-term antihypertensive treatment. J Hypertens 1995;13:1091-105.
8. Levy D, Salomon M, D'agostino RB, Belanger AJ, Kannel WB. Prognostic implications of baseline electrocardiographic features and their serial changes in subjects with left ventricular hypertrophy. Circulation 1994;90:1786-93.
9. Fragola PV, Colivicchi F, Fabrizi E, Borzi M, Cannata D. Assessment of left ventricular hypertrophy in patients with essential hypertension. A rational basis for the electrocardiogram. Am J Hypertens 1993;6:164-9.
10. Kannel WB. Prevalence and natural history of electrocardiographic left ventricular hypertrophy. Am J Med 1983;75:4-11.
11. Reichek N, Devereux RB. Left ventricular hypertrophy: relationship of anatomic, echocardiographic and electrocardiographic findings. Circulation 1981;63:1391-8.
12. Devereux RB, Casale PN, Wallerson DC, et al. Cost effectiveness of echocardiography and electrocardiography for detection of left ventricular hypertrophy in patients with systemic hypertension. Hypertension 1987;9(pt.2):II69-76.
13. Woythaler JN, Singer SL, Kwan OL, et al. Accuracy of echocardiography versus electrocardiography in detecting left ventricular hypertrophy:comparison with postmortem mass measurements. J Am Coll Cardiol 1983;2:305-11.
14. Kannel WB. Hypertension, hypertrophy and the occurrence of cardiovascular disease. Am J Med Sci 1991;302:199-204.
15. Casale PN, Devereux RB, Milner M, et al. Value of echocardiographic measurement of left ventricular mass in predicting cardiovascular morbid events in hypertensive men. Ann Intern Med 1986;105:173-8.
16. Levy D, Garrison RJ, Savage DD, Kannel WB, Castelli WP. Prognostic implications of echocardiographically determined left ventricular mass in the Framingham Heart Study. N Engl J Med 1990;322:1561-6.
17. Reichek N. Standardization in the measurement of left ventricular wall mass. Two-dimensional echocardiography. Hypertension 1987;9(2pt.2):II30-2.
18. Kucherer HF, Kuebler WW. Diagnosis of left ventricular hypertrophy by echocardiography. J Cardiovasc Pharmacol 1992;19:S81-6.
19. Weiss JL, McGaughey M, Guier WH. Geometric considerations in determination of left ventricular mass by two-dimensional echocardiography. Hypertension 1987;9(Suppl II):II85-9.
20. Sahn DJ, DeMaria A, Kisslo J, Weyman A. The Committee on M-Mode Standardization of the American Society of Echocardiography: Recommendations regarding quantitation in M-mode echocardiography: results of a survey of echocardiographic measurements. Circulation 1978;58:1072-83.
21. Devereux RB, Reichek N. Echocardiographic determination of left ventricular mass in men. Anatomic validation of the method. Circulation 1977;55:613-8.
22. Teicholz LE, Kreulen T, Herman MZ, Gorlin R. Problems in echocardiographic volume determinations: echocardiographic-angiographic correlations in the presence or absence of asynergy. Am J Cardiol

1976;37:7-11.

23. Missouris CG, Forbat SM, Singer DRJ, Markandu ND, Underwood R, MacGregor GA. Echocardiography overestimates left ventricular mass: a comparative study with magnetic resonance imaging in patients with hypertension J Hypertens 1996 14:1005-10.

24. Devereux RB, Alonso DR, Lutas EM, et al. Echocardiographic assessment of left ventricular hypertrophy: comparison to necropsy findings. Am J Cardiol 1986;57:50-8.

25. Wikstrand J. Calculation of left ventricular mass in man-a comment. 1997;15:811-3.

26. Rackley CE, Dodge HR, Coble YD, Hay RE. A method for determining left ventricular mass in man. Circulation 1964;29:666-71.

27. Troy BL, Pombo J, Rackley CE. Measurement of left ventricular wall thickness and mass by echocardiography. Circulation 1972;45:602-11.

28. Schillachi G, Verdecchia P, Porcelatti C. Does echocardiography overestimate ventricular mass? [letter] J Hypertens 1997;15:213-4.

29. Missouris CG, Forbat SM, Singer DRJ, Markandu ND, Underwood R, MacGregor GA. Does echocardiography overestimate left ventricular mass? [letter] J Hypertens 1997;15:213.

30. Ganau A, Devereux RB, Roman MJ, et al. Patterns of left ventricular hypertrophy and geometric remodeling in essential hypertension. J Am Coll Cardiol 1992;19:1550-8.

31. Schnellbaecher MJ, Gopal AS, Shen Z, Akinboboye OO, Sapin PM, King DL. Human in vitro validation using explanted hearts: superior accuracy of 3D echo over 2D and 1D echo for left ventricular mass determination. [abstract] Circulation 1995;92(Suppl):1-803.

32. Just H, Holubarsch C, Friedburg H, Estimation of left ventricular volume and mass by magnetic resonance imaging: comparison with quantitative biplane angiocardiography. [abstract] Cardiovasc Intervent Radiol 1987;10:1A.

33. Allison JD, Flickinger FW, Wright JC, et al. Measurement of left ventricular mass in hypertrophic cardiomyopathy using RI: comparison with echocardiography. Magn Reson Imaging 1993;11:329

34. Maddahi J, Creus J, Berman DS, et al. Noninvasive quantification of left ventricular myocardial mass by gated proton nuclear magnetic resonance imaging. J Am Coll Cardiol 1987;10:682-92.

35. Shapiro EP, Rogers WJ, Beyar R, et al. Determination of left ventricular mass by magnetic resonance imaging in hearts deformed by acute infarction. Circulation 1989;79:706-11.

36. Mogelvang J, Lindvig K, Sondergaard L, Saunamaki K, Henriksen O. Reproducibility of cardiac volume measurements including left ventricular mass determined by MRI. Clin Physiol 1993;13:587-97.

37. Matheijssen NAAM, Baur LHB, Reiber JHC et al. Assessment of left ventricular volume and mass by cine magnetic resonance imaging in patients with anterior myocardial infarction:intra-observer and inter-observer variability on contour detection. Int J Card Imaging 1996;12:11-9.

38. Germain P, Roul G, Kastler B, Mossard JM, Bareiss P, Sacrez A. Inter-study variability in left ventricular mass measurement. Comparison between M-mode echocardiography and MRI. Eur Heart J 1992;13:1011-9.

39. Baur LHB, Schipperheyn JJ, van der Velde EA et al. Reproducibility of left ventricular size, shape and mass with echocardiography, magnetic resonance imaging and radionuclide angiography in patients with anterior wall infarction. Int J Card Imag 1996;12:233-40.

40. Aurigemma G, Davidoff A, Silver K, Boehmer J. Left ventricular mass quantitation using single-phase magnetic resonance imaging. Am J Cardiol 1992;70:259-62.

41. Vogel M, Stern H, Bauer R, Buhlmeyer K. Comparison of magnetic resonance imaging with cross sectional echocardiography in the assessment of left ventricular mass in children without heart disease and in aortic isthmic coarctation. Am J Cardiol 1992;69:941-4.

42. Turpeinen A, Kuikka J, Vanninen E et al. Athletic heart:a metabolic, anatomical and functional study. Med Sci Sports Exerc 1996;28:33-40.

43. Pluim BM, Beyerbacht HP, Chin JC et al. Comparison of echocardiography with magnetic resonance imaging in the assessment of the athlete's heart. Eur Heart J 1997;18:1505-13.

44. Collins HW, Kronenberg MW, Byrd BF III. Reproducibility of left ventricular mass measurements by two-dimensional and M-mode echocardiography. J Am Coll Cardiol 1989;14:672-6.

45. Fast J, Jacobs S. Limits of reproducibility of cross-sectional echocardiographic measurements of left ventricular muscle mass. Int J Cardiol 1991;31:213-6.

46. Gardin JM, Siscovick D, Anton-Culver H et al. Sex, age and disease affect left ventricular mass and systolic function in the free living elderly: The cardiovascular health study. Circulation 1995;91:1739-48.

47. Harregods M, De Paep G, Bijnens B et al. Determination of left ventricular volume by two-dimensional echocardiography:comparison with magnetic resonance imaging. Eur Heart J 1994;15:1070-3.

48. Friedman B, Waters J, Kwan O, Demaria A. Comparison of magnetic resonance imaging and echocardiography in determination of cardiac dimensions in normal subjects. J Am Coll Cardiol 1985;5:1369-76.

49. Helbing W, Bosch H, Maliepaard C et al. Comparison of echocardiographic methods with magnetic

resonance imaging for assessment of right ventricular function in children. Am J Cardiol 1995;76:589-94.

50. Bottini PB, Carr AA, Prisant LM, Flickinger FW, Allison JD, Gottdiener JS. Magnetic resonance Imaging compared to echocardiography to assess left ventricular mass in the hypertensive patient. Am J Hypertens 1995;8:221-8.
51. Okin PM, Roman MJ, Devereux RB, Borer JS, Kligfield P. Electrocardiographic diagnosis of left ventricular hypertrophy by the time-voltage integral of the QRS complex. J Am Coll Cardiol 1994;23:133-40.
52. Lavie CJ jr., Nunez BD, Garavaglia GE Messerli FH, Hypertensive concentric left ventricular hypertrophy: when is ventricular ectopic activity increased? South Med J 1988;81:696-700.
53. Kannel WB, The clinical heterogeneity of hypertension. Am J Hypertens 1991;4:283-7.
54. Aronow WS, Epstein S, Koenigsberg M, Schwartz KS. Usefulness of echocardiographic left ventricular hypertrophy, ventricular tachycardia and complex ventricular arrhythmias in predicting ventricular fibrillation or sudden cardiac death in elderly patients. Am J Cardiol 1988;62:1124-5.
55. Devereux RB, Pini, R, Aurigemma GP, Roman MJ. Measurement of left ventricular mass: methodology and expertise. J Hypertens 1997;15:801-9.

5. HYPERTROPHY AND HYPERTENSION

J.J. SCHIPPERHEIJN

Summary

All types of muscle adapt to a sustained load by increasing the thickness of their fibres. Heart muscle adapts to the high wall stress caused by hypertension by increasing the mass of the left ventricle. As a result, the heart in hypertensives operates, due to an increase in thickness of only a few millimetres, at an only moderately increased level of wall stress. Because of the cubic relationship between ventricular dimensions and volume, ventricular mass is nevertheless considerably increased. The mechanism of ventricular hypertrophy is stimulation of protein synthesis by force development, mediated by the concentration of free calcium ions in the sarcoplasma. Cardiac hypertrophy induces sooner or later a process of down-regulation of cellular function and repair processes that eventually leads to accelerated cell death and cardiac failure. Hypertension is the main cause of cardiac failure.

Introduction

Hypertrophy of heart muscle is modified by humoral factors. Angiotensin-II, endothelin and noradrenaline have considerable influence on protein synthesis, either by modulating the activity of stress-activated protein kinases or by affecting intracellular calcium concentrations. Hypertrophy is modified as well by the properties of contractile proteins and by the handling of calcium ions by the sarcoplasmatic reticulum. Inhibition of the calcium pump of the sarcoplasmatic reticulum increases the intracellular concentration of calcium ions in the muscle cells and, as a result, promotes development of hypertrophy. Nitric oxide stimulates the uptake of calcium ions into the sarcoplasmatic reticulum and inhibits hypertrophy. Loss of endothelial function in patients with hypertension and hyperlipidemia is therefore expected to stimulate development of hypertrophy. Treatment of hyperlipidemia improves endothelial function. It has been shown that, as a result of improved endothelial function, life expectancy in cardiac

E. E. van der Wall et al.(eds.), Left Ventricular Hypertrophy, 55-64.
© 1999 *Kluwer Academic Publishers. Printed in the Netherlands.*

failure is increased. Similar to the treatment with angiotensin converting enzyme (ACE)-inhibitors and ß-adrenoreceptor blockers, this is probably due to inhibition of hypertrophy which delays development of heart failure.

Hypertension is the most common cause of hypertrophy of the left ventricle and subsequently of heart failure. Hypertension is a cardiovascular risk factor, but the risk is greatly enhanced if hypertension is accompanied by hypertrophy. It is important to look into the mechanisms that determine the slope of the relationship between blood pressure and cardiac muscle mass. Medical treatment of hypertension lowers the risk, but in case cardiac muscle mass is increased, treatment should be aimed not only at lowering the blood pressure, but also at reducing ventricular hypertrophy. Regression of hypertrophy reduces the associated additional risk and prevents development of heart failure.

Load adaptation

If heavy loads are imposed upon a muscle regularly and for an extended period of time, all the muscle fibres increase in diameter and muscle mass increases. This is a universal property of muscle, found in mammals, birds, fishes and even in insects. It is present in all types of muscle; in skeletal and cardiac muscle the cells only grow in size, in smooth muscle the cells increase in size as well as in number.

Due to load adaptation, the wall thickness of the left ventricle increases in patients in whom systolic ventricular pressure is raised continuously because of hypertension or aortic valve stenosis. Wall thickness increases also in patients suffering from hypertrophic cardiomyopathy in whom force development in the heart muscle is compromised, while systolic pressure inside the ventricle is normal. Apparently, it is load relative to the capacity to develop force that stimulates growth. As in muscle there exists a reciprocal relationship between force development and velocity of fibre shortening, stimulation of protein synthesis by force development and inhibition by fibre shortening is therefore a fundamental property of muscle. It seems most likely, that the concentration of free calcium ions in the vicinity of the myofibrils acts as the signal that links force development to protein synthesis.

Apart from its ability to adapt to pressure load, the heart is able to dilate in case volume load is increased permanently. Adaptation to volume load, which implies passive stretching of muscle fibres is unique to the heart. In skeletal muscles passive stretch is not possible due to the bones to which the muscles are attached. Dilation primarily involves the connective tissue of the heart not present in other muscles. In manual labourers, professional dancers and athletes, but also in patients with chronic anemia, mitral or aortic valve incompetence, or with hearts damaged by infarction or some other disease process, the left ventricle dilates. Dilation involves disruption and subsequent reattachment of collagen tethers that connect imbricating layers of fibre bundles. A rise in filling pressure, i.e. mean left ventricular diastolic pressure, maintained for a sufficiently long period of time, is all that is needed to stretch the heart muscle. Just like other structures, like ear lobes and lips, that are kept in shape by connective tissue, the heart yields to passive stretch, provided it is maintained long enough.

Because of the Laplace relation of diameter, wall thickness and wall stress, dilation of the heart raises wall stress even when systolic pressure remains unchanged. Wall stress is raised additionally because dilation causes thinning of the wall. Dilation is therefore a powerful stimulus for hypertrophy of the muscle. In fact the largest values of ventricular muscle mass are found in hearts adapted to large volume loads, as in patients with aortic valve incompetence. Dilation and hypertrophy are therefore linked together and are often referred to in a single word as remodeling. There is no dilation without hypertrophy and hypertrophy without any dilation is possible but rare. Even in hypertension where high systolic pressure primarily induces the hypertrophy that reduces wall stress, the ventricle dilates. Hypertrophy lowers wall stress, but not to the level found in normotensives. The enddiastolic dimensions increase slightly and due to Starling's mechanism the heart muscle is able to generate the remaining wall stress.

Load sensitivity of contractile protein synthesis in muscle is a well conserved property in the evolution of species and the essential parts of the genes involved must have been conserved for several hundred million years. Loss or damage of those genes apparently reduces the chances of survival considerably, because there appear to be no species that have survived without it. The adaptation to load is therefore a 'physiological' property; physiological in the sense of normal, healthy and appropriate. The process is fully reversible. When load is reduced and the muscle develops less stress, muscle mass returns to its original value. The same is true for adaptive dilation of the heart. As soon as filling pressure is reduced, by surgical repair of valve incompetence for instance, the size of the heart returns to normal.

Hypertrophy of the heart muscle involves cellular growth regulating mechanisms that appear to be governed by the intracellular concentration of calcium ions. Apart from the hemodynamic load, hormonal factors also exert strong influences on protein synthesis, probably mainly by modulating sarcoplasmatic concentrations of calcium ions. Noradrenaline, angiotensin II and endothelin not only have a short-term positive inotropic action, but also a long-term stimulating effect on protein synthesis.

Scientists involved in culturing heart muscle cells found that passive stretch of the cells promotes growth. It is likely, that due to the length-dependent affinity of troponin for calcium ions, passive stretch leads to an increased binding of calcium ions, which acts as a stimulus for protein synthesis. Stretch-induced hypertrophy, however, is also mediated in these cells by an autocrine and paracrine release of growth-promoting substances like angiotensin-II, endothelin and ATP.[1]

It is not clear how development of stress stimulates protein synthesis, but is likely that calcium ions play an important role. If blood pressure is high, the heart muscle is not able to shorten properly. As a result, the binding of calcium ions to troponin is prolonged. This will increase the concentration of calcium ions, which may act as the signal that stimulates protein synthesis. The stretch-induced release of growth promoting hormones promote the influx of calcium ions and as a result raise intracellular calcium levels. In that way they promote protein synthesis.

Wall stretch and stress

The concentration of calcium ions is certainly not the only trigger for protein synthesis. More recent research in this field has revealed that stretch, as well as stress development, have a direct influence on the activity of G-proteins involved in the expression of genes for the synthesis of contractile proteins.[2,3] Nevertheless, there are a number of pathways along which cell growth can be stimulated, and calcium ions play a key role in all of them.

In the heart, the number of cells does not increase after birth, the contractile proteins within the cells, however, are continuously renewed. From the time-course of regression of hypertrophy after surgical treatment of aortic valve stenosis, or of the time course of development of compensatory hypertrophy after a large myocardial infarction, the time constant of protein turnover can be estimated at about 100 days, both for increase and decrease. Relative to the life span of heart muscle cells, protein turnover is rapid. This implies that the rate of protein synthesis has to remain above normal, to maintain the hypertrophy. Since wall stress is the stimulus for protein synthesis, wall stress has to stay elevated in hypertrophic heart muscle. However, wall stress is inversely proportional to wall thickness and hypertrophy of the heart muscle thus reduces wall stress. The development of ventricular hypertrophy is therefore under feed-back control. If a person develops hypertension, the wall stress in the left ventricle increases and cardiac muscle cells grow in size, until wall stress is normalized. In practice, wall stress has to remain at a moderately elevated level to keep protein synthesis permanently at the higher level required to sustain hypertrophy. In hypertensives, left ventricular mass is higher than normal and despite the greater wall thickness, wall stress is always elevated. Hypertrophy in hypertension reduces excess wall stress for only about 50 percent. The remaining excess in wall stress acts as an error signal that maintains protein synthesis at a permanently elevated level. Suppose, systolic pressure in the heart is normally 120 mmHg and wall thickness is 9 mm. Suppose, hypertension develops and systolic pressure increases to 160 mm Hg permanently. Wall stress, as a result, increases with 33% and wall thickness has to increase to 12 mm to fully normalize wall stress. Because of some ventricular dilation, wall thickness must increase even more, up to 13 mm for full normalization, that is by 44%. On average, however, wall thickness in persons with a permanently elevated systolic blood pressure of 160 mmHg measures only about 11 mm, which means that a 33% increase in systolic blood pressure leads to a 22% increase in wall thickness and a wall stress that remains 22% higher than normal despite compensatory hypertrophy. Because of the cubic relationship between wall thickness and volume, left ventricular mass, however, is increased by more than 80%. Compensatory dilation of the heart is also under feed-back control. If filling pressure is raised, the heart increases in size until stroke volume is sufficiently increased to accommodate the volume load and to lower the filling pressure and diastolic stretch sufficiently to stop further dilation. Like in control of hypertrophy the enddiastolic stretch of the ventricle is maintained at a moderately elevated level.

Modulation of hypertrophy

Heart muscle hypertrophy, for any given level of stress, is modulated by hormones, growth factors and in extreme cases even by oxygen supply and metabolism.[45] Cardiac muscle mass rarely exceeds twice the normal value. There are experimental data that show that hormonal influences may regulate protein synthesis upwards, as well as downwards. Upward regulation leads to excessive hypertrophy up to the limits set by the metabolism of the muscle fibres.

Downward regulation reduces contractility and promotes cell death and leads to cardiac failure. Downward regulation without sufficient hypertrophy results in a dilating cardiomyopathy. Excessive upward regulation leads to an extreme form of ventricular hypertrophy like in hypertrophic cardiomyopathy. Upward regulation may on the long term turn into downregulation. How compensatory hypertrophy turns into failure is probably the most important question at the moment in this field of research. Why does downward regulation begin so early in some patients, while others live with extreme hypertrophy to over the age of 80. This issue is of great importance for the management of patients with hypertension. Some of them show only moderate compensatory hypertrophy until old age and never go into failure. Others show excessive hypertrophy at an early age and go into failure 40 or 50 years of age. It would be very important to know how the growth promoting and growth reducing mechanisms can be controlled.

Stimulation of type 1 angiotensinereceptors for angiotensin-II (AT_1-receptors), of α-adrenergic receptors for noradrenaline ($α_1$-receptors) and for endothelin (ET-receptors) all initially promote the development of hypertrophy. The effect of stimulation of these receptors is mediated by a number of stress-activated protein kinases. Genetic abnormalities in the chain of factors involved in the regulation of protein synthesis by these hormones may have a considerable effect on the degree of hypertrophy.[6] Many studies on protein synthesis in experimentally induced hypertrophy have shown that all hypertrophic muscle cells eventually express, to some extent, proteins that reduce contractile function, inhibit protein synthesis and cause cardiac failure. Among many other phenomena there is down-regulation of adrenergic receptors, promotion of the synthesis of foetal forms of myosin, reduction of the affinity of troponin for calcium ions, reduced expression of ryanodine receptors and inhibition of the uptake of calcium ions into the sarcoplasmatic reticulum, and induction of cytoskeletal changes that create a viscous load and impair contractile function.[7] Eventually, these changes induce apoptosis and reduce muscle mass.[8] Some of these mechanisms are clearly protective in the sense that they protect the muscle cell from excessive stimulation by hormones that may threaten metabolic supply or may cause mechanical damage. Most of the mechanisms, however, are deleterious, as they induce cardiac failure and decrease life expectancy. Research in this field should be aimed at finding ways to block down-regulation as soon as it becomes deleterious. Inhibition of the type 1 angiotensin-II receptor, or the adrenergic receptor reduces hypertrophy and delays the development of failure, whereas contractility is not impaired. This suggests that long-lasting and excessive humoral stimulation of protein synthesis and the hypertrophy itself eventually induces heart failure and not the wall stress.

Calcium turnover

New insights into the mechanism of compensatory hypertrophy have come from the study of the calcium turnover in heart muscle and its effect on muscle mass. During the action potential a small quantity of calcium ions enters the cell and releases more calcium ions from the sarcoplasmatic reticulum (SR). The calcium sensitive receptor on the SR that triggers Ca^{++} release is called the ryanodine receptor (RyR). The SR contains a calcium-binding protein called calsequestrin (CS). Calcium ions released from the SR bind to troponin and initiate the contraction. At the end of the contraction, calcium ions are released from troponin and are pumped back into the SR by a calcium-sensitive ATP-ase, or calcium pump, called SERCA-2. The SERCA-2 activity is carefully regulated. It is inhibited by phospholambam (PLb); upregulation of SERCA-2 activity is possible by reducing the inhibitory activity of PLb by phosphorylation. Phosphorylation of PLb by cyclic guanylmonophosphate (cGMP) is in fact upregulation of calcium uptake by desinhibition of SERCA-2. Noradrenaline does the same, through cyclic adenylmonophosphate (cAMP) it causes desinhibition of SERCA-2 which improves the uptake of calcium ions and shortens relaxation.

By genetic techniques the influences of practically all factors involved in calcium turnover on development of hypertrophy have been studied. In general, all interventions that compromise the uptake or the release of calcium ions from the SR induce hypertrophy. As a result of such interventions, less calcium ions are available from the SR for binding to troponin, contractile function is impaired and fibre shortening is reduced. To compensate for the reduction of the number of calcium ions from the SR, the affinity of troponin for calcium ions is increased by stretching the fibre, by phosphorylation of troponin and, in addition, contractility is restored by increasing the influx of calcium ions into the cell. This results in higher intracellular concentrations of Ca^{++} ions while the calcium turnover by the SR is reduced. As a result, the synthesis of new myofibrils is stimulated by the calcium ions. Hypertrophy thus provides the long-term solution to the problem of SR dysfunction.

The PLb knock-out mouse lacks the usual inhibitory influence of PLb on SERCA-2. As a result the SR stores calcium ions more effectively than usual, contractility is enhanced and development of hypertrophy is somewhat depressed.[9] With genetically manipulated PLb that is not phosphorylatable the reverse happens.[10] It strongly inhibits SERCA-2, reduces calcium uptake and promotes development of hypertrophy. Intoxication or genetically induced malfunction of the RyR,[11] overexpression of CS,[12] or inhibition of SERCA-2 all reduce contractile function, but promote the development of hypertrophy.

The phosphorylation of PLb, which reduces its inhibitory influence on SERCA-2, reduces hypertrophy by counteracting inhibition. Phospholamban is phosphorylated by cyclic GMP that is formed under the influence of NO. This accounts for the inhibitory effect of nitrates on ventricular hypertrophy, while loss of endothelial function promotes the development of hypertrophy. Hyperlipidemia, hypertension and diabetes, which are known to compromise endothelial function, can by this mechanism promote hypertrophy of the left ventricle.

Clinical implications

In patients with long-standing hypertension left ventricular mass is always increased, but not always to the same extent.[13] The correlation between mean systolic pressure and mass is usually weak. This is partly due to measurement errors in the assessment of both blood pressure and mass, but polymorphism of genes regulating the many growth factors involved, and of the properties of contractile proteins and calcium turnover in the SR play a significant role. This follows from studies on the heritability of left ventricular hypertrophy. The slope of the relationship between systolic pressure and left ventricular mass therefore varies from person to person. Left ventricular hypertrophy is said to be an independent risk factor, but it is in fact the slope of the pressure-mass relationship that determines prognosis independently from blood pressure. For any degree of hypertension, mortality from hypertrophy-induced heart failure or arrhythmias is increased proportional to left ventricular mass. Left ventricular hypertrophy is in fact target organ damage that, if it occurs, complicates hypertension and greatly increases mortality. According to the latest report of the Joint National Committee[14] even persons with a high-normal blood pressure above 135/85 mmHg and target organ damage should be treated medically to reduce the risk. The high risk of left ventricular hypertrophy makes it worth while to do so. The limit for medical treatment for uncomplicated hypertension according to the report remains at 160/100 mmHg, but for hypertensives with left ventricular hypertrophy 135/85 mmHg should be the criterium.

Target of the treatment of hypertension with left ventricular hypertrophy is reduction of blood pressure to a completely normal level. The results of the large HOT[15] trial has demonstrated that the target of treatment should be the complete normalization of the blood pressure. If left ventricular mass is increased treatment should be aimed at additionally reducing excessive cardiac muscle mass and delaying development of heart failure by inhibiting the receptors involved. Treatment of hypertension with left ventricular hypertrophy is pharmacologically the same as treatment of heart failure in normotensive patients. In hypertensive patients with left ventricular hypertrophy the risk of going into cardiac failure is considered to be as high as in patients with normal or reduced wall thickness and a left ventricular ejection fraction below 40%. Because of the increased wall thickness, ejection fraction greatly overestimates contractile function in hypertensives and it cannot be used as a proper criterium for heart failure. As inhibition of the type 1 angiotensin and adrenergic receptors delays development of heart failure in normotensives, it is likely to do so in hypertensives with left ventricular hypertrophy.

Conclusions

Many hypertensive patients develop coronary artery disease. Hypertension compromises endothelial integrity which promotes the development of plaques. Patients with combined hyperlipidemia often have hypertension. In hypertensive patients with hypercholesterolemia left ventricular mass seems to be larger than in other hypertensives. Results from basic research indicate that poor endothelial function caused by hyperlipidemia promotes the development of ventricular hypertrophy. As explained above, the mechanism involved may be insufficient stimulation of SERCA-2 by nitric oxide. Recently published data from the 4S-trial[16] in which patients with coronary artery disease were treated with simvastatine, show that in a subset of patients with heart failure, treatment of the hyperlipidemia delays development of heart failure and reduces mortality from progression of failure. This demonstrates the importance of treating patients with hypertension and left ventricular hypertrophy not simply with any blood pressure lowering drug, but with agents that block all mechanisms that reduce hypertrophy. This may include treatment that protects endothelial function.

References

1.   Uozumi H, Kudoh S, Zou Y, Harada K, Yamazaki T, Komuro I. Autocrine release of ATP mediates mechanical stress-induced cardiomyocyte hypertrophy. [abstract] Circulation 1998;98(Suppl 1):624.
2.   Aikawa R, Zou Y, Tanaka M, Yamazaki T, Komura I. Rho family of small G proteins mediates mechanical stress-induced hypertrophic responses in cardiac myocytes. [abstract] Circulation 1998(Suppl 1);98:623.
3.   Choukroun G, Hajjar R, Rosenzweig A, Force T. The stress-activated protein kinases mediate cardiac hypertrophy. [abstract] Circulation 1998(Suppl 1);98:68.
4.   Zhang J, Gong G, Murakami Y, Zhang Y, Ye Y. Myocardial creatine kinase and contractile reserve in hearts with severe LV remodeling. [abstract] Circulation 1998(Suppl 1);98:419.
5.   Horn M, Remkes H, De Groot M, Hu K, Ingwall JS. Severe phosphocreatine depletion by beta-guanidinoproprionate increases mortality and aggravates hypertrophy in rats after myocardial infarction. [abstract] Circulation 1998(Suppl 1);98:538-9.
6.   Bella JN, MacCluer J, Roman MJ, et al. Heritability of left ventricular dimensions and mass: The Strong Heart Study. [abstract] Circulation 1998(Suppl 1);98:658.
7.   Zile MR, Green R, Schuyler GT, Aurigemma G, Miller C, Cooper G 4th. Mechanisms causing myocardial failure in man: Cytoskeletal changes in patients with pressure overload hypertrophy (POH). [abstract] Circulation 1998(Suppl 1);98:361-2.
8.   Bo D, Ma L, Weinberg EO et al. Aortic stenosis mice with LV hypertrophy: Apoptosis and transition to early failure. [abstract] Circulation 1998(Suppl 1);98:346.
9.   Sato Y, Yamamoto S, Yatani A, Kranias EG. Rescue of the depressed contractile parameters in calsequestrin overexpressing hearts by phopholamban ablation. [abstract] Circulation 1998(Suppl 1);98:53.
10. Brittsan AG, Kadambi VJ, Hoit BD, Kranias EG. Cardiac overexpression of a non-phosphorylatable form of phospholamban results in depressed contractile function and hypertrophy. [abstract] Circulation 1998(Suppl 1);98:490.
11. Hittinger L, Ghaleh B, Chen JK et al. Reduced ryanodine receptors and effects of ryanodine on cardiac function in dogs with severe left ventricular hypertrophy. [abstract] Circulation 1998(Suppl 1);98:489.
12. Knollmann BC, Duc J, Groth A, Weissman NJ, Cleemann L, Morad M. Cardiac phenotype of transgenic mice overexpressing calsequestrin. [abstract] Circulation 1998(Suppl 1);98:490.
13. Boekhout I, Van Marwijk HWJ, Petri H et al. Incidenteel verhoogde bloeddruk in de huisartspraktijk: bij meer dan de helft van de patiënten hypertensie en of linkerventrikelhypertrofie. Ned Tijdschr Geneeskd 1998;142:2404-8.
14. The sixth report of the Joint National Committee on prevention, detection, evaluation, and treatment of high blood pressure. Arch Intern Med 1997;157:2413-46.
15. Hansson L, Zanchetti A, Carruthers SG et al. Effects of intensive blood-pressure lowering and low-dose aspirin in patients with hypertension: principal results of the Hypertension Optimal Treatment (HOT) randomised trial. Lancet 1998;351:1755-62.
16. Kjekshus J, Pedersen TR, Olsson AG et al. The effects of simvastatin on the incidence of heart failure in patients with coronary heart disease. J Card Fail 1997;3:249-54.

6.   LEFT VENTRICULAR HYPERTROPHY:
PATHOLOGY VERSUS PHYSIOLOGY

B.M. PLUIM, A. VAN DER LAARSE, H.W. VLIEGEN,
A.V.G. BRUSCHKE, E. E. VAN DER WALL

Summary

Because of the increased risk for adverse cardiac events it is important to differentiate between physiologic (exercise-induced) and pathologic (disease-induced) left ventricular hypertrophy. Physiologic hypertrophy usually occurs in highly-trained athletes and can be considered as a normal adaptation to a chronic pressure or volume overload. Pathologic left ventricular hypertrophy is the result of maladaptation of the heart to overload and is a strong risk factor for cardiovascular morbidity and sudden death. Pathologic left ventricular hypertrophy may be congenital (e.g. hypertrophic cardiomyopathy) or acquired (e.g. hypertension). The main focus of this chapter is hypertension-induced left ventricular hypertrophy. Hypertension is the most common cause of left ventricular hypertrophy in the general population, which is associated with diastolic function abnormalities and an increased incidence of ventricular arrhythmias. Regression of left ventricular hypertrophy by antihypertensive drugs [e.g. angiotensin converting enzyme (ACE)-inhibitors] has been associated with lower cardiac mortality and improved prognosis of cardiovascular events. In addition to morphological changes, other criteria such as diastolic function, proneness to rhythm disturbances, family history and the electrocardiogram can be used to classify an enlarged heart as either a physiological or a pathological phenomenon.

Introduction

Left ventricular hypertrophy is the result of adaptation of the heart to a chronic pressure or volume overload, or the result of the influence of neurohumoral factors such as 1) increased circulating catecholamines, 2) increased discharge of cardiac sympathetic nerves, 3)

E. E. van der Wall et al.(eds.), Left Ventricular Hypertrophy, 65-84.
© 1999 *Kluwer Academic Publishers. Printed in the Netherlands.*

activation of the renin-angiotensin-aldosterone system, 4) increased levels of thyroxine, and 5) increased levels of growth hormone.[1-3] The hypertrophy consists of an increase in the volume of cardiac myocytes (hypertrophy) due to changes in diameter, length and volume, and an increase in the number of nonmuscle cells (hyperplasia). Pathologic left ventricular hypertrophy is an unfavorable prognostic sign and has gained wide recognition as an important independent risk factor for sudden death, ventricular arrhythmias, myocardial ischemia, and congestive heart failure.[4]

In this chapter, the assessment, prevalence, mortality, pathophysiology, geometry, function, electrocardiography, and regression of left ventricular hypertrophy are discussed in relation to physiological and pathological hypertrophy. As physiological hypertrophy usually occurs in highly trained athletes, which will be described in a next chapter, the main focus of this chapter will be on pathologic left ventricular hypertrophy due to hypertensive heart disease. This is because 1) hypertension is the most common cause of left ventricular hypertrophy in the general population, and 2) the hemodynamic load of the heart during exercise mostly resembles the hemodynamic load of the heart due to hypertension.

Assessment of left ventricular hypertrophy

Detection of left ventricular hypertrophy by electrocardiography, chest x-ray, echocardiography or magnetic resonance imaging is based on the ability of these techniques to demonstrate structural and fuctional changes and on the use of appropriate reference values.[5] Left ventricular hypertrophy is detected in about 10 times more subjects by echocardiography than by electrocardiography in the same population when the Framingham criteria for electrocardiographic left ventricular hypertrophy are used.[6] Thus, the correlation between electrocardiographic and echocardiographic left ventricular mass is weak (closest correlation 0.48), with a sensitivity ranging from 12 to 34% and a specificity ranging from 82 to 100%.[7] The poor correlation between the anatomical and electrocardiographic diagnosis of left ventricular hypertrophy suggests that they may be reflecting different phenomena.[8,9] It is generally assumed that the greater the increase in left ventricular mass, the higher the voltages that can be recorded on the electrocardiogram. However, chamber dilatation seems to play a greater role than wall thickening in augmenting surface potentials, which may explain part of the absence of a correlation between echocardiographic and electrocardiographic left ventricular hypertrophy.[10] It has been hypothesized that the ST-T segment changes on the electrocardiogram do not reflect an increase in left ventricular mass, but dysfunction of myocardial cells.[9] Electrocardiography is therefore not suitable for an accurate screening of left ventricular hypertrophy. However, once electrocardiographic left ventricular hypertrophy is present, it has a high predictive value for morbidity and mortality. Therefore, and because of its wide availability, electrocardiography should keep its place in the diagnosis of left ventricular hypertrophy. Echocardiography, on the other hand, has important limitations arising from the two-dimensional nature of the technique, particularly in subjects with an abnormal left ventricular geometry.[11]

Magnetic resonance imaging, a technique that has - independent of left ventricular geometry - a good reproducibility and accuracy in the quantification of left ventricular mass, is a suitable alternative to echocardiography as a reference method.[12] However, because of the low cost, easy applicability and wide availability of echocardiography, calculation of the left ventricular mass by echocardiography is the most widely used reference method for quantifying left ventricular hypertrophy. The advantages and limitations of the different measures to detect left ventricular hypertrophy are discussed in Chapter 4 by Brees.

A clear consensus concerning left ventricular hypertrophy cut-off values has not yet been achieved,[13] although all available studies agree that left ventricular mass should be indexed by using body size parameters, of which body surface area is most widely used.[5] Another issue is the use of gender-specific criteria, since the prevalence in men and women may differ depending on the use of gender-specific or gender-independent criteria. When a single cut-off value is used (120 g/m^2), the prevalence of left ventricular hypertrophy is consistently higher among hypertensive men (26 to 56%) than among hypertensive women (18 to 42%).[5] However, when gender-specific criteria are used, a higher proportion of female (43 to 61%) than male (18 to 41%) hypertensives exhibit left ventricular hypertrophy.[5] The generally used gender-specific echocardiographic cut-off values are 110 g/m^2 for women and 134 g/m^2 for men, representing the 97th percentile of values in apparently normal subjects.[5]

Predisposing factors and prevalence

Correlates of left ventricular mass include age, blood pressure, exercise, coronary and valvular heart disease, smoking, and body size.[14] The prevalence of left ventricular hypertrophy increases progressively with age. In the Framingham population, left ventricular hypertrophy was detected by echocardiography in 3 to 7% of adults under 50 years of age, and in 12 to 40% of individuals between 50 and 80 years of age.[15] This probably relates to increasing weight and blood pressure with age, since the association between age and left ventricular mass or wall thickness disappears after adjusting for systolic blood pressure and body mass index.[16] There is a positive relation between body weight and left ventricular mass, with a 9-fold (women) to 10-fold (men) increase in prevalence of left ventricular hypertrophy from leanest to most obese subjects.[15,17] In the Treatment Of Mild Hypertension Study (TOMHS), a weight loss of 4.5 kg in 3 months was associated with an 8 g loss in left ventricular mass.[18]

Hypertension

The most common cause of left ventricular hypertrophy in the general population is hypertension.[19] For each increment of 10 mmHg in mean systolic pressure, left ventricular mass index increases by about 20 g/m^2.[20] Left ventricular hypertrophy has been demonstrated by echocardiography in 13 to 26% of patients with mild hypertension.[16,21] Although hypertension is a major cause of left ventricular hypertrophy, clinical studies show rather poor correlations between left ventricular mass and casual blood pressure readings.[22] Only 6 to 20% of the variance in left ventricular mass can be explained by casual blood pressure readings,[23] 20 to 35% by 24-hour ambulatory blood pressure,[24] 15 to 35% by blood pressure readings during regularly recurring stress,[25] and 8 to 12% by the lack of a nocturnal blood pressure decline.[26]

Hence, it has been suggested that in addition to hemodynamic load, non-mechanical factors may be involved in the development of left ventricular hypertrophy in hypertension. Genetic influences, including ACE gene polymorphism, have been shown to influence left ventricular mass.[27,28] Carriers of the ACE genotype with two deletion alleles (DD-genotype), associated with increased ACE-levels in plasma, have a 4-fold increased risk of left ventricular hypertrophy (in the absence of hypertension) than carriers with the deletion/insertion allele (ID-genotype) or two insertion alleles (II-genotype).

Both angiotensin-II, aldosterone, β_1-adrenoreceptor agonists, endothelin-1, and bradykinin appear to affect cardiac size independent of blood pressure.[3,28,29] The greater reversal of left ventricular hypertrophy for a given fall in blood pressure with ACE-inhibitors compared to other antihypertensive drugs is consistent with this pressure-independent effect mediated by the renin-angiotensin-aldosterone system.[30] In Chapter 10 by Van der Laarse the efficacy of ACE-inhibitors in reversal of left ventricular hypertrophy is extensively described.

Mortality

Left ventricular hypertrophy is a powerful risk factor for a variety of cardiovascular disease sequelae, including angina pectoris, myocardial infarction, stroke, congestive heart failure, and sudden death.[8] In echocardiographic left ventricular hypertrophy, the relative risk of sudden cardiac death is 1.70 for every 50 g/m increment in left ventricular mass indexed to height.[31] Electrocardiographic left ventricular hypertrophy, particularly when accompanied by repolarization abnormalities, is associated with pronounced excess mortality when compared to echocardiographic or x-ray determined cardiac enlargement without electrocardiographic changes,[6,8] and cardiovascular risk increases substantially and proportionally to the severity of voltage and repolarization abnormalities.[32] Left ventricular hypertrophy with repolarization abnormalities ("strain" pattern) is associated with 59% mortality over 12 years, whereas a left ventricular pattern based on voltage criteria alone, has a 16% mortality over 12 years.[6] Left ventricular mass is a stronger risk factor for cardiovascular events in women than in men.[15,19] In the elderly, the impact of left ventricular hypertrophy on mortality is greater than in younger subjects.[6] The pathophysiological mechanisms underlying the increased cardiovascular mortality in left ventricular hypertrophy may be 1) impaired diastolic and systolic function,[33] 2) reduced coronary vasodilator reserve,[34] and 3) ventricular arrhythmias.[35]

Pathophysiology

Ventricular hypertrophy may be considered as 1) hypertrophy of cardiac myocytes due to increments in diameter, length and volume, and 2) hyperplasia of nonmuscle cells, in response to a chronic increase in wall stress or in response to neurohumoral factors.[1,2,29] According to Laplace's law, the degree of left ventricular wall stress is directly proportional to the intracavitary pressure and the radius of the chamber, and is inversely proportional to wall thickness.[4,36] Thickening of the myocardial wall therefore reduces wall stress. The type of cardiac overload determines the pattern of hypertrophy, i.e. concentric versus eccentric hypertrophy.

Pressure overload

Pressure overload, such as a sustained increase in mean arterial pressure, leads to an increase in the hemodynamic load of the left ventricle. Thus, stroke work, wall stress and myocardial oxygen consumption increase in response to pressure load. The heart adapts to these changes by adding contractile elements in parallel to thicken the left ventricular wall, associated with reduction of wall stress (Figure 1).[37]

Since chamber volume is unaffected, the relative wall thickness (posterior wall thickness divided by radius of the chamber) increases. This form of left ventricular hypertrophy is referred to as concentric left ventricular hypertrophy; in other words thickening of the wall is accompanied by an unchanged chamber volume.

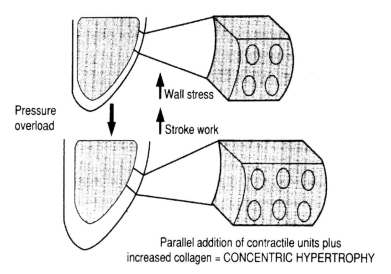

Figure 1. *In pressure overload, the ventricle enlarges by addition of sarcomeres in parallel, leading to increased ventricular wall thickness. The size of the ventricular cavity is unchanged or reduced. This is called concentric hypertrophy. From Struijker Boudier et al. Cardioreparation, CBC Oxford, Oxford, 1993, page 13. Reprinted with permission.*

Volume overload

Volume overload due to, for example, mitral valve insufficiency, leads to an increase in end-diastolic chamber volume and radius. In the fully compensatory stage, volume overload is associated with an increase of absolute left ventricular wall thickness that is proportional to the increase in left ventricular chamber radius, resulting in an unchanged relative wall thickness.[38] This situation, in which the mass increases away from the central axis of the ventricle, is called eccentric hypertrophy. The contractile elements are added in series as well as in parallel (Figure 2).

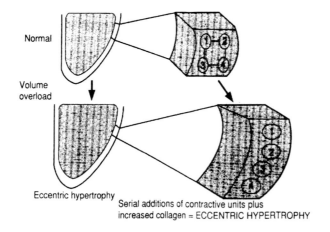

Figure 2. *In volume overload, the ventricle enlarges by addition of sarcomeres in series, leading to enlargement of the ventricular cavity without thickening of the left ventricular wall. This is called eccentric hypertrophy. From Struijker Boudier et al. Cardioreparation, CBC Oxford, Oxford, 1993, page 13. Reprinted with permission.*

Hyperplasia

Hypertrophy of the myocardium includes not only hypertrophy of myocytes, but also hyperplasia of nonmuscle cells such as fibroblasts, vascular smooth muscle cells, endothelial cells, and increased concentrations of fibrillar collagen.[39] Factors other than hemodynamic load influence the degree of cardiac fibrosis, including angiotensin 2, β_1-adrenoreceptor agonists, aldosterone, endothelin-1, and bradykinin.[29] The inappropriate increase in collagen content has been shown to be a major contributing factor to the development of a reduced coronary vasodilator reserve and reduced ventricular compliance.[40]

Coronary flow reserve

Reduced coronary reserve develops when growth of the coronary bed is not in proportion to the increase in cardiac mass, resulting in decreased capillary density and an increased diffusion distance.[2,41] Even though the total myocardial blood flow in left ventricular hypertrophy is increased, the blood flow per gram of tissue may be reduced.[42]

In compensated hypertrophy the endocardial/epicardial flow ratio and the relation between endocardial blood supply and demand are normal, whereas the coronary flow reserve is attenuated. When left ventricular pump failure develop, the endocardial/epicardial flow ratio and the relation between supply and demand are marginal and there is hardly any flow reserve. Such conditions are likely to lead to episodic subendocardial ischemia during periods of hemodynamic stress. Recurrent subendocardial ischemia results in biochemical adjustments and eventually myocardial necrosis, cell loss, and fibrosis which would exacerbate left ventricular dysfunction. This sequence of events characterizes the transition from compensated hypertrophy to cardiac failure.

Anatomic structure and dimensions

Although one might expect that patients with high blood pressure would uniformly develop concentric left ventricular hypertrophy to an extent proportional to the level of blood pressure, several studies indicate that this is not the case.[43] Left ventricular geometric adaptation to hypertension is complex, and generally three types of structural changes can be distinguished: concentric left ventricular hypertrophy (increased mass and increased relative wall thickness), *concentric* remodeling (normal mass and increased relative wall thickness), and *eccentric* left ventricular hypertrophy (increased mass and normal relative wall thickness) (Figure 3).[43,44]

Ganau et al.[43] demonstrated that cardiac geometric adaptation matches systemic hemodynamic and ventricular load. Concentric remodeling occurs when there is an *increased* peripheral resistance and *reduced* cardiac index, with high resting blood pressure. Eccentric hypertrophy, on the other hand, occurs as a result of a *normal* total peripheral resistance and *high* cardiac index, with increased resting blood pressure. Concentric hypertrophy is related to a *normal* cardiac index, *elevated* total peripheral resistance, and the *highest* level of blood pressure.

The pattern of left ventricular hypertrophy may modulate the risk of cardiovascular events.[19] Subjects with concentric hypertrophy have the highest risk, those with normal geometry have the lowest risk, and subjects with eccentric hypertrophy or concentric remodeling have an intermediate risk for adverse cardiac events. For any given value of left ventricular mass, the risk associated with concentric remodeling in the presence of normal left ventricular mass, or with concentric hypertrophy in the presence of increased left ventricular mass, is higher by 1 to 1.5 major events per 100 patient-years than the risk associated with normal left ventricular geometry or eccentric hypertrophy, respectively.[45]

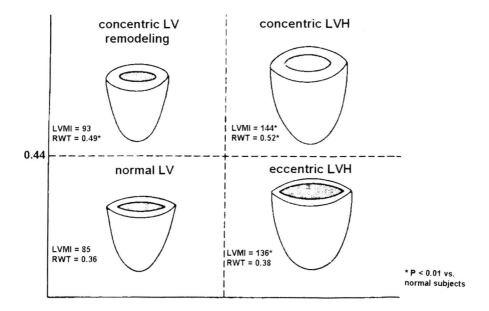

Figure 3. The four patterns of left ventricular geometry in hypertensive patients. LVMI indicates left ventricular mass index; RWT indicates relative wall thickness. From Ganau et al. J Am Coll Cardiol 1992;19:1550-1558. Reprinted with permission (ref.65).

Myocardial function

Systolic function

Left ventricular systolic function is generally assessed by 1) measuring the extent and velocity of fiber shortening, i.e. ejection fraction and velocity of circumferential fiber shortening, and by 2) relating these parameters to systolic wall stress. A normal relation between left ventricular ejection fraction (or fractional shortening) and wall stress is usually preserved in patients with hypertensive left ventricular hypertrophy until late in the course of the disease.[4,38] However, the parameters used in whole heart studies reflect chamber mechanics, not myocardial mechanics. Studies of myocardial contractile function in the hypertrophied left ventricle suggest that intrinsic myocardial performance may be depressed in hypertensive left ventricular hypertrophy, even though the left ventricular ejection fraction is normal.[46] In cases with borderline changes, examination during physical stress (exercise testing) may provoke a decrease in left ventricular systolic function, due to an exercise-induced oxygen supply/demand imbalance.[47] The deterioration in systolic function will eventually lead to ventricular dilatation and congestive heart failure. These patients with so-called systolic heart failure will have reduced left ventricular ejection fraction.

Diastolic function

Diastole involves the time period from aortic valve closure to mitral valve closure. Diastolic function is commonly assessed by studying the pattern of ventricular filling through the mitral valve.[48] Diastolic function abnormalities, characterized by impaired diastolic filling of the left ventricle, generally occur earlier in the course of the disease than systolic dysfunction.[33] In some hypertensive patients, diastolic filling abnormalities correlate significantly with left ventricular mass and wall thickness,[33,49] but abnormal left ventricular filling has also been observed in the absence of hypertrophy.[50] Impaired left ventricular filling observed in patients with left ventricular hypertrophy results from both a prolonged early diastolic relaxation and a diminished late diastolic compliance.[51] Although increased left ventricular mass can influence chamber stiffness through simple geometric mechanisms, myocardial fibrosis may contribute by virtue of an influence on intrinsic myocardial stiffness.[52] Angiotensin-II, aldosterone, norepinephrine, and endothelin-1 stimulate myocardial fibroblasts, leading to increased synthesis of extracellular matrix components and a consequent increase in myocardial tissue stiffness in hypertensive left ventricular hypertrophy.[29] Delayed or incomplete relaxation due to myocardial ischemia may cause additional stiffening.[51]

Electrocardiographic changes in left ventricular hypertrophy

Electrocardiographic abnormalities have been described in left ventricular hypertrophy since the early days of the electrocardiogram. Some 33 electrocardiographic criteria for left ventricular hypertrophy have been reported.[53] The increased amplitude of the QRS complex is the basis of most criteria for left ventricular hypertrophy (i.e. voltage criteria).[42] In the Framingham study, electrocardiographic left ventricular hypertrophy was diagnosed when at least one of the following voltage criteria was met: R wave >1.1 mV in aVL; R wave >2.5 mV in V5 or V6; S wave > 2.5 mV in V1 or V2; sum of S wave in V1 or V2 plus R wave in V5 or V6 >3.5 mV; or sum of R wave in I and S wave in III >2.5 mV.[32] Repolarization was categorized as normal, mildly abnormal (ST-T flattening, isolated ST depression, or T-wave inversion) or severely abnormal (left ventricular strain pattern, i.e. ST depression in association with inverted or biphasic T waves) (Figure 4). However, sensitivity of the Framingham criterion for left ventricular hypertrophy is very low (9%).[7] Another commonly used method to diagnose left ventricular hypertrophy is the Romhilt-Estes point-score system,[54] that incorporates information about the QRS amplitude, the ST-T segment, left atrial involvement, left axis deviation, QRS duration, and intrinsicoid deflection (Table I). The authors[54] claimed a sensitivity to diagnose left ventricular hypertrophy of 60% for their point-score system, but in the study of Schillaci et al.[7] comprising 923 patients, a much lower sensitivity of only 18% was found. The newly developed scoring system presented in the latter study[7] incorporates three different criteria and is very promising. It includes the Romhilt-Estes score as well as the Cornell voltages (sum of the amplitudes of the S wave in V3 and the R wave in aVL with different partition values for males and females) and left ventricular strain. The scoring system has a sensitivity of 34% and a specificity of 93%.[7]

Ventricular arrhythmias

It has been shown that left ventricular hypertrophy is associated with an increased incidence of ventricular arrhythmias.[31,35,55,56] The question has been raised whether the frequency and complexity of ventricular arrhythmias in hypertensive patients might be markers for sudden cardiac death, as in almost all monitored cases, sudden death is caused

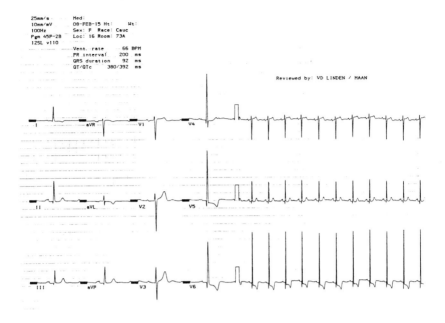

Figure 4. Electrocardiographic left ventricular hypertrophy with strain pattern. SV1 and RV5 = 4.6 mV. ST segment depression and asymmetrical T wave inversion in V5 and V6.

by ventricular fibrillation and ventricular tachycardia.[31,35,56] Indeed, in the study by Bikkina et al.,[57] the presence of asymptomatic ventricular arrhythmias in subjects with left ventricular hypertrophy was associated with a high mortality, which remained statistically significant after adjusting for age, gender, body mass index, blood pressure, cholesterol, smoking, diabetes, therapeutic drug use, and congestive heart failure. Various mechanisms have been put forward to explain the presence of ventricular arrhythmias in hypertensive patients with left ventricular hypertrophy. Possible mechanisms are 1) abnormal membrane properties of hypertrophied myocytes, 2) conduction disturbances due to increased fibrous tissue, and 3) reduced coronary vascular reserve and silent myocardial ischemia.[57] Overload-induced hypertrophy of the cardiac myocyte is associated with several electrophysiological changes, such as an increase in the duration of the action potential, a decrease in the effective membrane capacity, and an increased susceptibility to triggered activity and arrhythmias.[58,59] Increased QT-dispersion, an index of nonhomogeneity of repolarization, has been demonstrated in patients with severe left ventricular hypertrophy. The resulting variations in conduction velocity could form the basis of a reentrant circuit in ventricular tachyarrhythmias.[60] Reduced coronary reserve and myocardial ischemia occur in

Table 1. Point-score system according to Romhilt-Estes[54]

	Points
1. Amplitude	3
Positive if any of the following are present:	
1) largest R or S wave in the limb leads ≥20 mm,	
2) S wave in V1 or V2 ≥30 mm,	
3) R wave in V5 or V6 ≥30 mm.	
2. ST-T segment	
without digitalis	3
with digitalis	(1)
Positive if typical ST-T strain pattern is present (ST-T segment	
vector shifted in opposite direction to mean QRS vector).	
3. Left atrial involvement	3
Positive if the terminal negativity of the P wave in V1 is 1	
mm or more in depth with a duration of ≥0.04 s	
4. Left axis deviation	2
Positive if left axis deviation of -30° or more is present	
in frontal plane	
5. QRS duration	1
Positive if QRS duration is ≥0.09 s	
6. Intrinsicoid deflection	1
Positive if intrinsicoid deflection in V5 or V6 ≥0.05 s	
Maximum total	13

Clarification of points

Three points or less	: no left ventricular hypertrophy
Four points	: probable left ventricular hypertrophy
Five points or more	: definite left ventricular hypertrophy

hypertensive left ventricular hypertrophy as a result of subendocardial perfusion abnormalities in the hypertrophied ventricle itself or from associated coronary artery disease.[41,61] The ischemic component may be arrhythmogenic. An increased incidence of arrhythmias has been shown to correlate with asymptomatic ST-T segment depression in normokalemic, untreated hypertensive subjects.[56]

Regression of left ventricular hypertrophy in hypertension

When left ventricular hypertrophy develops in the course of hypertension or ischemic heart disease, it should be regarded as a serious prognostic sign rather than an innocent compensatory phenomenon. Reversal of hypertrophy seems to be a logical therapeutic goal, since regression of left ventricular hypertrophy has been associated with lower cardiac mortality and an improved prognosis of cardiovascular events.[42,62] Interventions that may regress left ventricular hypertrophy include blood pressure control, weight loss, alcohol moderation in susceptible patients, and salt reduction.[18,63] Already after 4 weeks of antihypertensive therapy reduction of left ventricular mass can be observed.[64] A recent meta-analysis of randomized, double-blind trials showed that after a mean treatment duration of 25 weeks, left ventricular mass had decreased by 13% during therapy with ACE- inhibitors, by 9% with calcium-antagonists, by 6% with β-blocking agents, and by 7% with diuretics.[30] The longer the duration of therapy and the greater the decrease in blood pressure, the more marked the decrease in left ventricular mass.[30] (See also Chapter 10 by Van der Laarse).

Differentiation between physiological and pathological hypertrophy

The differential diagnosis between exercise-induced left ventricular hypertrophy and disease-induced pathologic left ventricular hypertrophy with the potential of sudden death is an important clinical problem. Such critical distinctions most commonly involve hypertrophic cardiomyopathy, myocarditis and hypertensive left ventricular hypertrophy. Hypertrophic cardiomyopathy is a primary myocardial abnormality with an autosomal dominant pattern of inheritance in which the characteristic gross morphologic abnormality is a hypertrophied (wall thickness ≥15 mm) and nondilated left ventricle, which exists in the absence of a coexisting cardiac or systemic disease that could induce left ventricular hypertrophy.[65] Acute myocarditis is an inflammatory process of the myocardium, often caused by viral infections.[66] Hypertensive hypertrophy is the pathologic left ventricular hypertrophy caused by arterial hypertension.[16,21] Echocardiographic studies have shown that in highly trained athletes left ventricular wall thickness may be substantially increased.[67] As a consequence, normal limits for diastolic wall thickness have been revised upwards, up to 16 mm (Figure 5).[67]

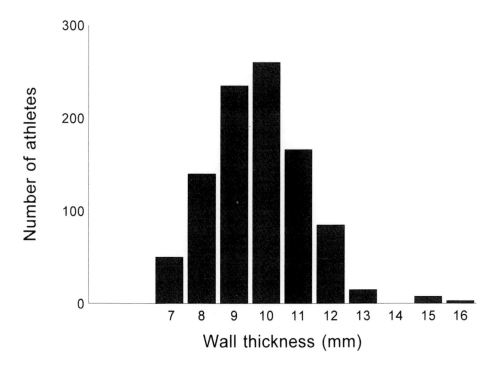

Figure 5. *Distribution of maximal left ventricular wall thickness in 947 elite athletes. From Pellicia et al. N Engl J Med 1991;324:295-301. Reprinted with permission. Copyright 1999 Massachusetts Medical Society. All Rights Reserved.*

These standards leave little margin of distinction between physiological hypertrophy and wall thicknesses of ≥15 mm that are typical of pathological forms of hypertrophy.[68] In the past, a ratio of the interventricular septum to posterior wall thickness >1.3 was considered to indicate pathology, but values >1.3 have been observed in athletes as well.[69,70] Thus, it is not possible to distinguish physiological and pathological hypertrophy on morphological criteria only.[71]

Additional criteria are needed to classify an enlarged heart as either an athlete's heart (physiologically enlarged) or a pathologically enlarged heart. The athlete's heart has to be distinguished from pathological conditions such as hypertension, hypertrophic cardiomyopathy and myocarditis. These criteria are summarized in Table 2.

Table 2. Differential diagnosis between the athlete's heart and hypertensive left ventricular hypertrophy, hypertrophic cardiomyopathy, and myocarditis.

	Athlete's heart[*]	Hypertensive LVH[**]	HCM[***]	Myocarditis[****]
Septum thickness (mm)	up to 19	↑	>13-15	n or ↓
Septum/post. wall ratio	n or >1.3	n or >1.3	>1.3	n
LV end-diastolic diameter (mm)	50 to 65	>45	< 45	>45
Relative LV wall thickness	n or ↑	n or ↑	↑	n or ↓
RV wall thickness	n	n	n	↓
RV dimension	n	n	n	↑
Diastolic function	n	n or ↓	↓	↓
Systolic function	n	n or ↓	n or ↑ or ↓	↑
Myocardial reflectivity	n	increased	increased	NR
LV biopsy	n	n or increased fibrosis	myocardial disarray	infiltrates; fibrosis
Family history	-	-	positive	-
Palpitations	-	n or ↑	↑	↑
(Supra)ventricular arrhythmias	-	↑	↑	↑
(Pre) syncope	-	-	↑	↑
Electrocardiogram	repolarization abnormalities	LVH, strain	inverted T waves	repolarization abnormalities, low voltage

↑ indicates increase; ↓ indicates decrease; n, the normal situation; HCM, hypertrophic cardiomyopathy; LV, left ventricular; LVH, left ventricular hypertrophy; NR, not reported; post., posterior; RV, right ventricular

* references 68,70,72-76
** references 33,51,57,74
*** references 65,72,75,78,79
**** references 66,77,78

Conclusions

Physiologic left ventricular hypertrophy should be clearly distinguished from pathologic hypertrophy as pathologic hypertrophy is a strong risk factor for a variety of cardiovascular disease sequelae, including angina pectoris, myocardial infarction, stroke, congestive heart failure, and sudden death. It is the result of adaptation of the heart to a chronic pressure or volume overload, including an increased neurohumoral activation. Hypertension is the most common cause of left ventricular hypertrophy in the general population. The pattern of left ventricular hypertrophy may modulate the risk of cardiovascular events, with subjects with concentric hypertrophy having the highest risk, those with normal geometry having the lowest risk, and subjects with eccentric hypertrophy or concentric remodeling having an intermediate risk for adverse cardiac events.

Mechanisms that have been put forward to explain the presence of ventricular arrhythmias in hypertensive left ventricular hypertrophy are 1) abnormal membrane properties of hypertrophied myocytes, 2) conduction disturbances due to increased fibrous tissue, and 3) reduced coronary vascular reserve and silent myocardial ischemia. Regression of left ventricular hypertrophy has been associated with lower cardiac mortality and improved prognosis of cardiovascular events. Because of the increased risk for adverse cardiac events it is important to differentiate between physiologic (exercise-induced) and pathologic (disease-induced) left ventricular hypertrophy. Therefore, the main differences between the physiologically enlarged heart and several types of pathologically enlarged hearts are outlined. It is shown that in addition to morphological changes, other criteria such as diastolic function, family history and the electrocardiogram can be used to classify an enlarged heart as either physiological or pathological.

References

1. Oparil S. Pathogenesis of left ventricular hypertrophy. J Am Coll Cardiol 1985;5:57-65.
2. Rapaport E. Pathophysiological basis of left ventricular hypertrophy. Eur Heart J 1982;3:29-33.
3. Weber KT, Sun Y, Guarda E. Structural remodeling in hypertensive heart disease and the role of hormones. Hypertension 1994;23:869-77.
4. Frohlich ED, Apstein C, Chobanian AV, et al. The heart in hypertension. N Engl J Med 1992;327:998-1008.
5. Devereux RB. Cardiac involvement in essential hypertension. Med Clin North Am 1987;71:813-26.
6. Kannel WB, Dannenberg AL, Levy D. Population implications of electrocardiographic left ventricular hypertrophy. Am J Cardiol 1987;60:85I-93I.
7. Schillaci G, Verdecchia P, Borgioni C, et al. Improved electrocardiographic diagnosis of left ventricular hypertrophy. Am J Cardiol 1994;74:714-9.
8. Kannel WB. Blood pressure as a cardiovascular risk factor. JAMA 1996;275:1571-6.
9. Dijkstra RF, Van Schayk CP, Bakx JC, Thien Th, Verheugt FWA, Mokkink HG. Linkerventrikelhypertrofie; verschillen in diagnostische en prognostische waarde van electrocardiografie en echocardiografie. Ned Tijdschr Geneeskd 1997;141:1969-72.
10. Kulbertus HE. Electrocardiographic aspects of left ventricular hypertrophy. In: Ter Keurs H, Schipperheijn J, editors. Cardiac left ventricular hypertrophy. Boston: Martinus Nijhoff Publishers, 1983. p. 197-207.
11. Allison JD, Flickinger FW, Wright JC, et al. Measurement of left ventricular mass in hypertrophic cardiomyopathy using MRI: comparison with echocardiography. Magn Reson Imaging 1993;11:329-34.
12. Sayad DE, GD Clarke, RM Peshock. Magnetic resonance imaging of the heart and its role in current cardiology. Curr Opin Cardiol 1995;10:640-9.
13. Abergel E, Tase M, Bohlender J, Menard J, Chatellier G. Which definition for echocardiographic left ventricular hypertrophy? Am J Cardiol 1995;75:498-502.
14. Gardin JM, Arnold A, Gottdiener JS, et al. Left ventricular mass in the elderly. Hypertension 1997;29:1095-103.
15. Levy D, Anderson KM, Savage DD, Kannel WB, Christiansen JC, Castelli WP. Echocardiographically detected left ventricular hypertrophy: prevalence and risk factors. The Framingham Heart Study. Ann Intern Med 1988;108:7-13.
16. Liebson PR, Grandits G, Prineas R, et al. Echocardiographic correlates of left ventricular structure among 844 mildly hypertensive men and women in the treatment of mild hypertension study (TOMHS). Circulation 1993;87:476-86.
17. Gottdiener JS, Reda DJ, Materson BJ, et al. Importance of obesity, race and age to the cardiac structural and functional effects of hypertension. J Am Coll Cardiol 1994;24:1492-8.
18. Liebson PR, Grandits GA, Dianzumba S, et al. Comparison of five antihypertensive monotherapies and placebo for change in left ventricular mass in patients receiving nutritional-hygienic therapy in the treatment of mild hypertension study (TOMHS). Circulation 1995;91:698-706.
19. Koren MJ, Devereux RB, Casale PN, Savage DD, Laragh JH. Relation of left ventricular mass and geometry to morbidity and mortality in uncomplicated essential hypertension. Ann Intern Med 1991;114:345-52.
20. Rowlands DB, Glover DR, Ireland MA, et al. Assessment of left ventricular mass and its response to antihypertensive treatment. Lancet 1982;1:467-70.
21. Hammond IW, Devereux RB, Alderman MH, et al. The prevalence and correlates of echocardiographic left ventricular hypertrophy among employed patients with uncomplicated hypertension. J Am Coll Cardiol 1986;7:639-50.
22. Fouad FM. Assessment of the function of the hypertrophied heart. In: Ter Keurs H, Schipperheyn J, editors. Cardiac left ventricular hypertrophy. Boston: Martinus Nijhoff Publishers; 1983. p. 115-28.
23. Drayer JIM, Weber MA, DeYoung JL. Blood pressure as determinant of left ventricular muscle mass. Arch Intern Med 1983;143:90-2.
24. Verdecchia P, Schillaci G, Boldrini F, et al. Risk stratification of left ventricular hypertrophy in systemic hypertension using noninvasive ambulatory blood pressure control. Am J Cardiol 1990;66:583-90.
25. Devereux RB, Pickering TG, Harshfield GA, et al . Left ventricular hypertrophy in patients with hypertension: importance of blood pressure response to regularly recurring stress. Circulation 1983;68:470-6.
26. Rizzo V, Piccirillo G, Cicconetti P, et al. Ambulatory blood pressure and echocardiographic left ventricular dimensions in elderly hypertensive subjects. Angiology 1996;47:981-9.
27. Schunkert H, Hense HW, Holmer SR, et al. Association between a deletion polymorphism of the angiotensin-converting-enzyme gene and left ventricular hypertrophy. N Engl J Med 1994;330:1634-8.
28. Harrap SB, Dominiczak AF, Fraser R, et al. Plasma angiotensin II, predisposition to hypertension, and left

ventricular size in healthy young adults. Circulation 1996;93:1148-54.

29. Susic D, Nunez E, Frohlich ED. Reversal of hypertrophy: an active biologic process. Curr Opin Cardiol 1995;10:466-72.

30. Schmieder RE, Martus P, Klingbeil A. Reversal of left ventricular hypertrophy in essential hypertension. JAMA 1996;275:1507-13.

31. Levy D, Garrison RJ, Savage DD, Kannel WB, Castelli WP. Prognostic implications of echocardiographically determined left ventricular mass in the Framingham Heart Study. N Engl J Med 1990;322:1561-6.

32. Levy D, Salomon M, D'Agostino RB, Belanger AJ, Kannel WB. Prognostic implications of baseline electrocardiographic features and their serial changes in subjects with left ventricular hypertrophy. Circulation 1994;90:1786-93.

33. Inouye I, Massie B, Loge BS, et al. Abnormal left ventricular filling: an early finding in mild to moderate systemic hypertension. Am J Cardiol 1984;53:120-6.

34. Vatner SF, Shannon R, Hittinger L. Reduced subendocardial coronary reserve. Circulation 1990;81:8-14.

35. McLenachan JM, Henderson E, Morris KI, Dargie HJ. Ventricular arrhythmias in patients with hypertensive left ventricular hypertrophy. N Engl J Med 1987;317:787-92.

36. Gaasch WH. Left ventricular radius to wall thickness ratio. Am J Cardiol 1979;43:1189-94.

37. Krayenbuehl HP, Hess O, Hirzel H. Pathophysiology of the hypertrophied heart in man. Eur Heart J 1982;3:125-31.

38. Devereux RB, Savage DS, Sachs I, Laragh JH. Relation of hemodynamic load to left ventricular hypertrophy and performance in hypertension. Am J Cardiol 1983;51:171-6.

39. Vliegen HW, Van der Laarse A, Cornelisse CJ, Eulderink F. Myocardial changes in pressure overload-induced left ventricular hypertrophy. Eur Heart J 1991;12:488-94.

40. Otterstad JE, Smiseth O, Kjeldsen SE. Hypertensive left ventricular hypertrophy: pathophysiology, assessment and treatment. Blood Press 1996;5:5-15.

41. Opherk D, Mall G, Zebe H, et al. Reduction of coronary reserve: a mechanism for angina pectoris in patients with arterial hypertension and normal coronary arteries. Circulation 1984;69:1-7.

42. Sloan PJM, Beevers DG. Hypertension and the heart. Eur Heart J 1983;4:215-22.

43. Ganau A, Devereux RB, Roman MJ, et al. Patterns of left ventricular hypertrophy and geometric remodeling in essential hypertension. J Am Coll Cardiol 1992;19:1550-8.

44. Savage DD, Garrison RJ, Kannel WB, et al. The spectrum of left ventricular hypertrophy in a general population sample: the Framingham study. Circulation 1987;75:26-33.

45. Verdecchia P, Schillaci G, Borgioni C, et al. Prognostic value of left ventricular mass and geometry in systemic hypertension with left ventricular hypertrophy. Am J Cardiol 1996;78:197-202.

46. Palmon L, Reichek N, Yeon SB, Clark NR, Browson D, Hoffman E, Axel L. Intramyocardial shortening in hypertensive left ventricular hypertrophy with normal pump function. Circulation 1994;89:122-31.

47. Hittinger L, Patrick T, Ihara T, et al. Exercise induces cardiac dysfunction in both moderate, compensated and severe hypertrophy. Circulation 1994;89:2219-31.

48. Nishimura RA, Housmans PR, Hatle LK, Tajik AJ. Assessment of diastolic function of the heart: background and current applications of Doppler echocardiography. Part 1: Physiologic and pathophysiologic features. Mayo Clin Proc 1989;64:71-81.

49. Fouad FM, Slominski JM, Tarazi RC. Left ventricular diastolic function in hypertension: relation to left ventricular mass and systolic function. J Am Coll Cardiol 1984;3:1500-6

50. Devereux RB, Pickering TG, Alderman MH, Chien S, Borer JS, Laragh JH. Left ventricular hypertrophy in hypertension: prevalance and relationship to pathophysiologic variables. Hypertension 1987;9:53-60.

51. Lorell BH, Grossman W. Cardiac hypertrophy: the consequences for diastole. J Am Coll Cardiol 1987;9:1189-93.

52. Stauffer JC, Gaasch WH. Recognition and treatment of left ventricular diastolic dysfunction. Prog Cardiovasc Dis 1990;32:319-32.

53. Romhilt DW, Bove KE, Norris RJ, et al. A critical appraisal of the electrocardiographic criteria for the diagnosis of left ventricular hypertrophy. Circulation 1969;40:185-95.

54. Romhilt DW, Estes EH. A point-score system for the ECG diagnosis of left ventricular hypertrophy. Am Heart J 1968;75:752-8.

55. Schillaci G, Verdecchia P, Borgioni C, et al. Association between persistent pressure overload and ventricular arrhythmias in essential hypertension. Hypertension 1996;28:284-9.

56. Zehender M, Meinertz T, Hohnloser S, et al. Prevalence of circadian variations and spontaneous variability of cardiac disorders and ECG changes suggestive of myocardial ischemia in systemic arterial hypertension. Circulation 1992;85:1808-15.

57. Bikkina M, Larson MG, Levy D. Asymptomatic ventricular arrhythmias and mortality risk in subjects with left ventricular hypertrophy. J Am Coll Cardiol 1993;22:1111-6.

58.   Aronson RS. Afterpotentials and triggered activity in hypertrophied myocardium from rats with renal hypertension. Circ Res 1981;48:720-7.

59.   Moalic JM, Charlemagne D, Mansier P, Chevalier B, Swynghedauw B. Cardiac hypertrophy and failure- a disease of adaptation. Modifications in membrane proteins provide a molecular basis for arrhythmogenicity. Circulation 1993; 87 (Suppl IV):21-6.

60.   Perkiömäki JS, Ikäheimo MJ, Pikkujämsä SM, et al. Dispersion of the QT interval and autonomic modulation of heart rate in hypertensive men with and without left ventricular hypertrophy. Hypertension 1996;28:16-21.

61.   Marcus ML, Koyanagi S, Harrison DG, Doty DB, Hiratzka LF, Eastham CL. Abnormalities in the coronary circulation that occur as a consequence of cardiac hypertrophy. Am J Med 1983;71:62-5.

62.   Muiesan ML, Salvetti M, Rizzoni D, Castellano M, Donato F, Agabiti-Rosei E. Assocation of change in left ventricular mass with prognosis during long-term antihypertensive treatment. J Hypertens 1995;13:1091-5.

63.   Jula AM, Karanko HM. Effects on left ventricular hypertrophy of long-term nonpharmacological treatment with sodium restriction in mild-to-moderate essential hypertension. Circulation 1994;89:1023-31.

64.   Schmieder R, Messerli FH, Sturgill D, Garavaglia GE, Nunez BD. Cardiac performance after reduction of myocardial hypertrophy. Am J Med 1989;87:22-7.

65.   Maron BJ, Bonow RO, Cannon RO, Leon MB, Epstein SE. Hypertrophic cardiomyopathy. Interrelations of clinical manifestations, pathophysiology, and therapy (second of two parts). N Engl J Med 1987;316:844-52.

66.   Karjalainen J, Heikkilä J, Nieminen MS, et al. Etiology of mild acute infectious myocarditis. Acta Med Scand 1983;213:65-73.

67.   Spirito P, Pellicia A, Proschan MA, et al. Morphology of the "athlete's heart" assessed by echocardiography in 947 elite athletes representing 27 sports. Am J Cardiol 1994;109:1038-44.

68.   Shephard RJ. The athlete's heart: is big beautiful? Br J Sports Med 1996;30:5-10.

69.   Menapace FJ, Hammer WJ, Ritzer TF, et al. left ventricular size in competitive weight lifters: an echocardiographic study. Med Sci Sports Exerc 1982;14:72-5.

70.   Douglas PS, O'Toole ML, Katz SE, Ginsburg GS. Left ventricular hypertrophy in athletes. Am J Cardiol 1997;80:1384-8.

71.   Staiger J, Drexler H, Dickhuth HH, Keul J. Zur Problematik der Wanddickenbestimmung (Echokardiographie, Autopsie) bei der Diagnose Herzhypertrophie. Pathologe 1988;9:158-63.

72.   Maron BJ. Structural features of the athlete heart as defined by echocardiography. J Am Coll Cardiol 1986;7:190-203.

73.   Kindermann W, Urhausen A. Das Sportherz und seine Abgrenzung. Fortschr Med 1991;109:33-6.

74.   Di Bello V, Pedrinelli R, Giorgi D, et al. Ultrasonic videodensitometric analysis of two different models of left ventricular hypertrophy. Hypertension 1997;29:937-44.

75.   Maron BJ, Pellicia A, Spirito P. Cardiac disease in young trained athletes: insights into methods for distinguishing athlete's heart from structural heart disease, with particular emphasis on hypertrophic cardiomyopathy. Circulation 1995;5:1596-601.

76.   Zeppilli P, Santini C, Palmieri V, Vannicelli R, Giordano A, Frustaci A. Role of myocarditis in athletes with minor arrhythmias and/or echocardiographic abnormalities. Chest 1994;106:373-80.

77.   Zeppilli P, Santinia C, Dello Russo A , Picani C, Giordano A, Frustaci A. Brief report: healed myocarditis as a cause of ventricular repolarization abnormalities in athlete's heart. Int J Sports Med 1997;18:213-6.

78.   Maron BJ, Bonow RO, Cannon RO, Leon MB, Epstein SE. Hypertrophic cardiomyopathy. Interrelation of clinical manifestations, pathophysiology, and therapy (first of two parts). N Engl J Med 1987;316:780-9.

79.   Lehmann M, Dickhuth HH, Dürr H, Gastmann U, Keul J. Zur Differentialdiagnose: physiologische-pathologische Hypertrophie des Herzens. Ein Fallbericht. Z Kardiol 1988;77:784-8.

7. THE ATHLETE'S HEART: A PHYSIOLOGICAL OR A PATHOLOGICAL PHENOMENON?

B.M. PLUIM, A. VAN DER LAARSE, E.E. VAN DER WALL

Summary

The term "athlete's heart" describes the heart of an athlete including all cardiovascular adaptations associated with long-term athletic training.[1,2] Characteristic findings observed in the majority of athletes are sinus bradycardia, increased left ventricular dimensions and mass, and well-defined electrocardiographic criteria for left ventricular hypertrophy.[1] Other common cardiac findings among athletes include midsystolic murmurs, audible third and fourth heart sounds, a variety of non-specific electrocardiographic abnormalities, and cardiomegaly on the chest x-ray.[3,4]

Historical perspective

The athlete's heart has been an intriguing issue to scientists for more than a century. One of the first descriptions of the athlete's heart was given by Osler in 1892, who compared the large hearts of athletes with those of race horses and greyhounds and raised the question of nature versus nurture by stating: *"The large heart of athletes may be due to the prolonged use of their muscles, but no man becomes a great runner or oarsman who has not naturally a capable if not a large heart"*.[5] The statement of Osler was followed by Henschen in 1898, who investigated enlargement of the heart in cross-country skiers by percussion of the chest.[6] Henschen started the debate on the nature of the athlete's heart by stating the question: "Är nu en förstoring af hjärtat konstaterad, så frågas: är den fysiologisk och gagnelig eller patologisk". (When an enlargement of the heart is found, the question is whether it is physiologic and beneficial, or pathologic). Henschen's conclusion was that the enlarged heart of athletes is a beneficial adaptation enabling the athlete to perform more

E. E. van der Wall et al.(eds.), Left Ventricular Hypertrophy, 85-106.
© 1999 *Kluwer Academic Publishers. Printed in the Netherlands.*

work. This point of view has since been challenged by scientists, who considered the athlete's heart a pathologically enlarged heart. In fact, there has never been as much controversy on any subject in sports medicine as on the interpretation of the athlete's heart. In the literature many different explanations for the pathologic basis of the athlete's heart can be found. The athlete's heart was thought to be caused by excessive strain resulting in acute myocardial failure,[7] by overexertion that exhausts the reserve strength of the heart,[8] by a preexisting weakness,[9] by a constitutional deficiency,[10] or by overexertion in a rheumatic, syphilitic, or congenitally damaged heart.[11] More recent arguments for pathologic hypertrophy in athletes are a high incidence of sudden cardiac death in high-level athletes,[12,13] a higher incidence than normal of lethal arrhythmias among athletes,[14,15] and the increased risk for sudden cardiac death associated with left ventricular hypertrophy in a general population.[16] Only the last argument, however, is supported by epidemiological data, which will be discussed in more detail below in the paragraph on sudden cardiac death.

Henschen[6] performed his investigation of the athlete's heart by using percussion. In later years the athlete's heart was characterized by chest X-radiography[7,17] or was inferred from well-defined electrocardiographic criteria for left ventricular hypertrophy.[18] With respect to chest radiography the work of Kjellberg et al.[19] is most interesting. They demonstrated a close relationship between cardiac volume and physical working capacity, with the larger hearts being able to perform more work. Further elaboration of this relation between cardiac volume and performance resulted in the development of the Nylin index (myocardial volume divided by stroke volume)[8] and the introduction of the maximum oxygen pulse (maximum oxygen uptake of the body per heart beat).[17] It was concluded that an increased Nylin index means that *"the reserve strength (of the heart) has been drawn upon in excess of the physiological limit"*,[8] whereas the increased oxygen pulse clearly demonstrated that the reserve capacity of the athlete's heart was not decreased but, in fact, increased.

Later, the radiographic information was combined with an examination of electrocardiographic voltages. Left ventricular hypertrophy was diagnosed if the sum of the S wave in V1 and the R wave in V5 exceeded 35 mm (3.5 mV), and right ventricular hypertrophy if the sum of the R wave in V1 and the S wave in V5 exceeded 10.5 mm (1.05 mV).[20,21] These and other criteria for left ventricular hypertrophy will be discussed in more detail in chapter two.

Anatomic data on the athlete's heart became available in 1935 and 1936 when Kirch et al.[22,23] reported findings of 35 athletes who experienced sudden death. In these studies a smooth transition from normally-sized hearts to strengthened hearts ("gekräftigt") and definite hypertrophy (12 endurance athletes) was demonstrated. Kirch et al.[22,23] emphasized that the term "athlete's heart" should only be used for those hearts with definite hypertrophy, either left-sided or right-sided. They considered these hearts to be healthy but hypertrophied as a result of physical exercise. Linzbach et al.[24] found a microscopic appearance of the athlete's myocardium that was identical to that of nonstressed myocardium. The terms "critical heart weight" and "critical ventricle weight" were introduced, indicating an upper limit to physiologic hypertrophy: 500 g for the total heart and 200 g for the left ventricle.[24] Beyond the critical heart weight, any increase would lead to myocardial deterioration. This concept was challenged by Dickhuth et al.[25] who proposed a relative heart weight of 7.5 g/kg body weight as the upper limit of normal, and a maximum relative left ventricular muscle mass of 3.5 g/kg. This interesting concept of a critical heart weight was used by Messerli et al.[26] to characterize the transition from left ventricular hypertrophy as an adaptive process to a disease state in patients with systemic hypertension. Even if the concept of a critical heart weight would be true in patients with pathologic left ventricular hypertrophy, to date there is no evidence that physiologic left ventricular hypertrophy in athletes may transform to a pathologic state over time.

Sudden cardiac death

Was the sudden death of the legendary Philippides who died in 490 B.C. after running from Marathon to Athens to announce the Greek Army's victory over the Persians caused by overexertion? Sudden death in well-recognized elite athletes often attracts substantial public attention and provokes public debate on the risks that are associated with heavy training and top level competition. Such a debate took place in the Netherlands when a total of 14 elite cyclists died suddenly in the period 1988-1990.[13] The question raised in this discussion was whether exercise-induced myocardial hypertrophy carries an increased risk for sudden cardiac death during extreme physical exertion such as performed during the "Tour de France". Arguments supporting the contention of an increased risk for sudden death in athletes include the assumed increased incidence of arrhythmias among athletes[14,15] and the increased risk for sudden cardiac death associated with left ventricular hypertrophy in the general population.[16,27] Epidemiological studies, however, do not support these arguments regarding presumed risk factors. In the majority of the studies a similar prevalence of either atrial or ventricular arrhythmias has been observed in athletes and untrained normal individuals.[28-30] In contrast, the study of Palatini et al.[31] demonstrated more complex ventricular arrhythmias in 40 long-distance runners compared to 40 sedentary control subjects. However, even if it is true that athletes have more frequent and complex arrhythmias than non-athletes (observed in only 1 out of 4 studies), this does not prove an increased risk for sudden cardiac death in athletes, since the long-term prognosis in asymptomatic healthy subjects with frequent and complex arrhythmias is similar to that of a healthy population.[32] In addition, lower morbidity and mortality, resulting in increased life expectancy, has been extensively documented in physically active subjects, both Olympic-level[33,34] and recreational-level athletes.[35-39] For example, Sarna et al.[34] demonstrated a mean life expectancy of 75.6 years in endurance-trained male athletes, 73.9 years in team athletes, and 71.5 years in strength-trained athletes vs. 69.9 years in the reference group, mainly explained by a decreased cardiovascular mortality. And even though most epidemiological studies do show an increased risk for sudden cardiac death during and immediately after exercise, this is compensated for by a decreased risk for sudden cardiac death with long term regular exercise.[36] At a low level of training, strenuous exercise is associated with a 56-fold risk of sudden cardiac death compared to exercise-free periods. In contrast, at a high level of training the risk of sudden cardiac death during peak exercise is elevated only fivefold, with an overall risk of cardiac arrest of only 40% of the risk of cardiac death of sedentary subjects.[36]

The current opinion is that the athlete's heart is not associated with an increased incidence of sudden cardiac death, in contrast to pathological left ventricular hypertrophy.[16] In most cases of sudden cardiac death in athletes there is a pathological condition underlying the incident.[40] This condition varies with respect to age. Athletes older than 35 years typically die of coronary artery disease, whereas the majority of those younger than 35 years die of structural, non-atherosclerotic heart disease.[41] The most common abnormalities in young athletes who die suddenly are hypertrophic cardiomyopathy, congenital coronary anomalies, right ventricular dysplasia, idiopathic concentric left ventricular hypertrophy, myocarditis, and Marfan's syndrome.[41-43] The risk of sudden cardiac death in young athletes is relatively low.[44] Epstein and Maron[44] estimated an incidence of 0.0005% per year (0.5 death per year per 100,000 participants), which is in agreement with the incidence found in healthy Air Force recruits (0.5 annual deaths per 100,000 participants during exercise).[45]

Pathophysiology

The normal heart adapts to an increased workload by growth. Hypertrophy is the principal response of the heart to overload from any cause, including physical exercise, hypertension, valvular heart disease or myocardial infarction, in order to normalize wall stress. According to the law of Laplace, wall stress is approximately proportional to the product of the intraventricular pressure and the ratio of the ventricular radius to wall thickness:

$$\text{Wall stress} = \text{Constant} \times \text{Pressure} \times \text{Radius} / \text{Wall thickness}$$

Two different patterns of myocyte growth can be distinguished: growth associated with addition of myofibrils in series (increase in chamber volume) and growth associated with addition of myofibrils in parallel (increase in wall thickness). The pattern of hypertrophy seems to be related to the type of overload. Volume overload associated with increased diastolic wall stress leads to the addition of sarcomeres in series and chamber enlargement (eccentric hypertrophy), whereas the pressure overload associated with increased systolic wall stress leads to parallel growth of sarcomeres and wall thickening (concentric hypertrophy).[46] Pressure per se or simply stretch of muscle fibers occurring with pressure or volume overload activates the genetic apparatus of the myocardial cell, resulting in enhanced synthesis of nucleic acid and proteins such as myosin.[47] Endurance-trained athletes who experience a large rise in cardiac output without large pressure loads are thus subject to volume load and eccentric hypertrophy, whereas strength-trained athletes who experience a marked rise in blood pressure with only a small increase in cardiac output develop concentric hypertrophy.

Anatomic structure and dimensions

Echocardiographic studies

A large number of longitudinal studies have shown that exercise training leads to increases in left ventricular dimensions and mass.[1,48,49] An average increase of 10% in left ventricular end-diastolic dimension, 15 to 20% in wall thickness, and 45% in left ventricular mass is found in athletes compared with control subjects matched for sex, age, and body size.[1] In addition, an increased left atrial size[50,51] and larger right ventricular dimensions[52,53] have regularly been shown in athletes as well.

Different sports have different impact on the heart.[2,49,54-56] It has been suggested that two types of athlete's heart exist: a strength-trained heart and an endurance-trained heart. This concept was introduced by Morganroth et al.[57] based on echocardiographic criteria. They proposed that athletes engaged in different types of exercise may develop different patterns of left ventricular hypertrophy. According to their theory, athletes involved in sports with a high dynamic component (e.g. running) develop predominantly an increase in left ventricular chamber size, with a proportional increase in wall thickness ("endurance-trained heart"), due to the volume overload associated with the high cardiac output characteristic for this type of exercise. As a consequence, the relationship between left ventricular wall thickness and left ventricular radius, i.e. the wall thickness/radius ratio, should not change in endurance-trained athletes. Athletes involved in mainly static or isometric exercise (e.g. weight-lifting) were assumed to develop predominantly increased left ventricular wall thickness with unchanged cardiac dimensions ("strength-trained heart"), caused by the pressure overload accompanying the high systemic arterial pressure characteristic for this type of exercise. Intra-arterial peak pressures exceeding 480/350 mm Hg have been measured during weight-lifting.[58] This should result in an increased wall thickness/radius ratio, i.e. an increased relative left ventricular wall thickness. Extensive review of all available literature shows a slightly increased relative wall thickness in endurance-trained athletes and a considerably increased relative wall thickness in strength-trained athletes (Figure 1). The majority of athletes will have an intermediate form of cardiac hypertrophy, since most sports include both static and dynamic components.[59]

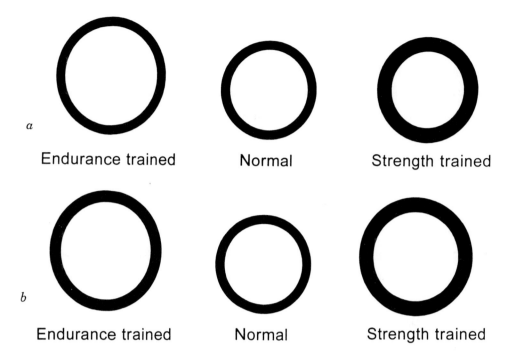

Figure 1a. Conventional representation of the anatomy of the athlete's heart as proposed in the literature: an endurance-trained heart with eccentric left ventricular hypertrophy and a strength-trained heart with concentric left ventricular hypertrophy.

Figure 1b. Representation of the athlete's heart according to our results; the classical concept of a great dichotomy between the endurance-trained and the strength-trained heart is challenged.

Female athletes

The cardiac morphology of female athletes is consistent with data reported for male athletes, but dimensions of the athlete's heart in women are generally smaller than those of the athlete's heart in men.[52,60] This is illustrated very well by a recent study of Pellicia at al,[60] who performed echocardiographic measurements in 600 elite female athletes and 65 sedentary female control subjects. Left ventricular cavity dimension, maximum wall thickness, and left ventricular mass index were higher in athletes compared to control subjects (by 6%, 14%, and 33%, respectively, all p<0.001). Compared with 738 previously studied male athletes, female athletes showed significantly smaller left ventricular cavity dimension, wall thickness, and left ventricular mass index (by 11%, 23%, and 33%, respectively, all p<0.001).

Magnetic resonance imaging studies

Relatively few studies on hearts of athletes have been performed using magnetic resonance techniques. Milliken et al.[61] were the first to use magnetic resonance imaging to measure left ventricular mass and left ventricular dimensions in athletes. Fleck et al.[62] found that weight-lifters had increased left ventricular wall thickness and increased diastolic internal dimensions. They found no effect of Olympic style weight-lifting upon the wall thickness or internal dimensions of the right ventricle. Riley-Hagan et al.[63] showed that female runners, cyclists, and cross-country skiers had increased left ventricular mass, volume, and mass to volume ratio. Pluim et al.

demonstrated prominent left ventricular hypertrophy and normal ventricular function and metabolism in cyclists, using magnetic resonance imaging and magnetic resonance spectroscopy (Figure 2).[64,65]

Myocardial function

The performance of the left ventricle as a pump depends on the contraction of the sarcomeres in the myocardium as well as the configuration of the left ventricular chamber and loading conditions. Cardiac function can thus be evaluated at several levels of integration: myocardial function, chamber (usually left ventricular) pump performance, and cardiac output.

Since it is not possible to measure absolute fiber length in the intact heart, cardiac function in athletes is usually evaluated by means of the systolic function parameters ejection fraction and fractional shortening, indication fractional changes in fiber length. However, since systolic function is a reflection of the interaction between loading conditions and contractility, it is important to take preload, afterload, heart rate and rhythm into account. Fractional shortening is the ratio of the difference between the end-diastolic (EDD) and end-systolic (ESD) diameter/end-diastolic diameter and is a measure of regional wall motion during systole. In formula: (EDD-ESD)/EDD.

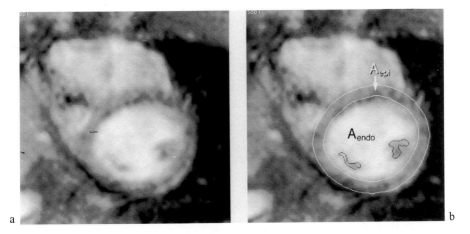

Figure 2a. Short-axis cine magnetic resonance images at mid-papillary level of a control subject (a) and a cyclist (b). The end-diastolic and end-systolic magnetic resonance images are shown. Note the increased left ventricular dimensions of the cyclist.

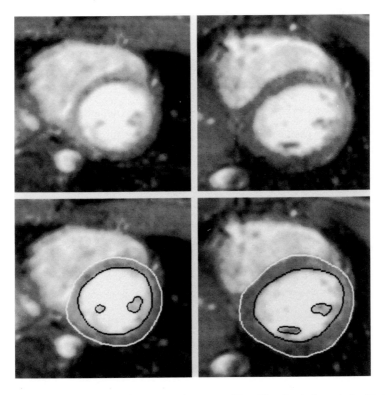

Figure 2b. Short-axis cardiac cine magnetic resonance images at mid-papillary level of a control subject (left), and cyclist (right). The end-diastolic magnetic resonance images without (upper panel) and with (lower panel) epicardial and endocardial contours are shown. Note the increased left ventricular dimensions of the cyclist.

Left ventricular ejection fraction or emptying fraction is the left ventricular stroke volume divided by the left ventricular end-diastolic volume. Left ventricular ejection fraction and fractional shortening in runners, cyclists or weight-lifers do not reveal any evidence of a significant effect of training on systolic left ventricular function with the possible exception of older elite cyclists.[66,67]

Normal diastolic left ventricular performance can be defined as the capacity to accept blood without a compensatory increase in left atrial pressure.[68] Diastolic dysfunction occurs when left ventricular filling is inadequate, incomplete or slow, resulting in abnormally high filling pressures in the left ventricle. The four major mechanisms that cause diastolic dysfunction are (1) abnormal myocardial relaxation, (2) pericardial restraint, (3) increased chamber stiffness, and (4) chamber dilatation.[69] Diastolic dysfunction has been shown to be an early consequence of pathologic left ventricular hypertrophy.[70,71] Several studies have shown that athletes with exercise-induced left ventricular hypertrophy have normal[72-74] or even slightly enhanced[75,76] diastolic properties of the left ventricle.

Myocardial function after exhaustive exercise

After extreme physical exertion such as 24 hour running, impairment of diastolic function (decreased E/A ratio) has been described.[77] Values return to normal after 2-3 days of rest. Impaired diastolic function after extreme exercise has been considered as a sign of cardiac fatigue, and it has been suggested to be comparable with myocardial stunning.[78,79] However, the fact that in untrained subjects less exercise duration causes a greater (transient) impairment of cardiac function substantiates the conclusion that cardiac fatigue after prolonged exercise is a normal finding, and not a sign of pathology.[80]

Electrophysiological changes in athletes

The electrocardiogram of highly trained athletes reflects the changes in the heart that have been brought about by training. The most common finding in athletes is resting bradycardia (heart rate less than 50 beats per minute).[81-82] In athletes the resting heart rate is generally 10 to 20 beats lower than in sedentary control subjects, but the heart rate can reach values as low as 21 beats per minute.[81] There is a positive association between the degree of bradycardia and the training state.[83] The mechanism of training-induced bradycardia at rest is the result of a lower intrinsic heart rate and an altered autonomic balance, i.e. an increased parasympathetic and a decreased sympathetic effect on the heart.[81,84]

Other electrophysiological findings, which are more common in athletes than in untrained individuals, are brady-arrhythmias such as sinus arrhythmia, first degree atrioventricular block, second degree atrioventricular block (type 1, Wenckebach), wandering atrial pacemaker, junctional rhythm and complete AV-block.[18,82,85] The sinus arrhythmia and conduction disturbances are probably secondary to the enhanced vagal tone due to training. During Valsalva maneuvers, atropine injection or exercise, normalization of the PQ interval occurs.[53,85] This also applies to the functional atrioventricular dissociation ("interference-dissociation") which may frequently be observed because of competition between junctional or idioventricular pacemakers and the sinus node (Figure 3).[86,87] During exercise, when the heart rate increases, the atrioventricular dissociation disappears and normal sinus rhythm resumes.[87,88] When a third degree atrioventricular block is present, underlying heart disease should be excluded by careful clinical examination.[85] The electrocardiographic changes mentioned above are not restricted to older athletes with many years of training; significant differences in sinus node function and atrioventricular conduction can also be found in prepubertal and teenage athletes.[89,90]

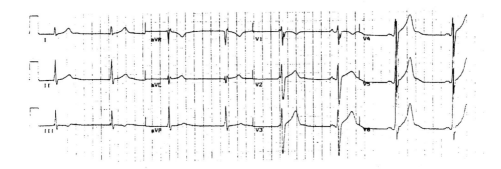

Figure 3. Atrioventricular dissociation at rest in the electrocardiogram of a 35-year old cyclist. This so-called "interference-dissociation" occurs because of competition between junctional pacemakers and the sinus node during sinus bradycardia.

The electrocardiograms of athletes often meet the criteria for left ventricular hypertrophy.[91] However, there is a poor correlation between electrocardiographic left ventricular hypertrophy and echocardiographic left ventricular mass, which may be due to the fact that the increased voltages not only reflect the increased cardiac mass but also the fact that most athletes are young and slim.[92]

It has been suggested that athletes might have a higher prevalence of atrial or ventricular arrhythmias, such as atrial or ventricular premature complexes, atrial fibrillation, or (supra)ventricular tachycardia than untrained individuals. However, with one exception,[31] there is no indication that the incidence of ventricular arrhythmias in athletes is increased in comparison to sedentary age-matched control subjects.[28-30] Talan et al.[28] performed 24 hour Holter analysis of 20 male long distance runners. Compared with 50 untrained males of similar age, the runners had the same prevalence of ventricular premature beats, ventricular couplets, or non-sustained ventricular tachycardia. These results were confirmed by Viitasalo et al.[29] in a study of 35 male athletes and 35 age-matched control subjects. Northcote et al.[30] observed an increased incidence of ventricular couplets and salvos in the 24-hour electrocardiograms of 21 highly trained squash players during and after training and competition compared to the resting situation, but the frequency was the same in an age-matched control group. The only study demonstrating a higher incidence of ventricular arrhythmias in athletes is that of Palatini et al.[31] They found no significant difference in the prevalence of ventricular ectopy between 40 athletes and 40 sedentary control subjects, but complex forms of ventricular ectopy were more prevalent among athletes than among control subjects (25% versus 5%).

The issue of an increased incidence of supraventricular arrhythmias is not fully resolved, due to a remarkable paucity of data and the absence of control groups in most studies.[93-94] The two studies that used control groups show opposite findings. Palatini et al.[31] found a similar prevalence of atrial arrhythmias in athletes and control subjects. Talan et al.[28] found an increased incidence of supraventricular ectopic beats (all athletes had at least one atrial premature beat versus 56% of controls) and atrial couplets (25% of athletes versus none of the controls). The prevalence of brief, nonsustained supraventricular tachycardia was similar in the two groups (10%).[28] There is no epidemiological evidence to substantiate the suggestion that atrial fibrillation is more common among athletes than among sedentary control subjects.[15,51]

P-wave changes consistent with right and left atrial overload have been observed in about half of the studies in athletes and represent right or left atrial enlargement.[95] The duration of the QRS complex is close to the upper limit of normal. Also, notching or slurring of the QRS complex in the right precordial leads or incomplete right bundle branch block are frequent findings among athletes (20 to 70%), as a result of right ventricular hypertrophy.[4,18] The QRS axis may be somewhat more vertical, but generally remains within normal limits.[3,18]

Ventricular repolarization abnormalities are fairly common in athletes, and different classification systems have been used in the past.[96] The most common findings are ST segment and J point elevation ("early repolarization"),[3,96] increased T wave amplitude,[3] persistent negative juvenile T wave patterns,[53] and prominent U wave voltages.[3] In a study of 1299 athletes and 151 sedentary control subjects ST elevations of more than 2 mm were found in 21.4% of athletes and 8.6% of control subjects (Figure 4).[3] A persistent juvenile T wave pattern (negative T waves from V1 to V4, generally of the terminal type) occurs with a frequency of up to 50% (Figure 5).[53] Negative T waves in V4 to V6, however, are relatively uncommon with a prevalence similar to that in the general population (0.4% versus 0.5%) and are more likely to indicate a pathologic state of the heart, particularly when associated with symmetric contour of T wave, ST segment depression, a prolonged QT interval, or absence of normal septal Q waves.[3,96] Also, QRS morphology of left bundle branch block and negative T waves in right precordial leads generally do not indicate an athlete's heart, but may raise suspicion of arrhythmogenic right ventricular dysplasia or myocarditis.[42]

The term heart rate variability refers to variations of both instantaneous heart rate and R-R interval length.[97] Changes in heart rate are primarily due to alterations in autonomic innervation of the sinus node, parasympathetic or vagal tone that slows heart rate, and sympathetic stimulation that increases heart rate. Exercise training results in increased parasympathetic activity at rest and is generally considered to lead to increased heart rate variability,[84,98,99] although some reports have failed to demonstrate such an increase.[100,101] The inconsistency in these results may partially be explained by the evaluation of young individuals who already have a high vagal tone, insufficient duration of the training program, intersubject variability, and cardiac sympathetic drive outlasting cessation of heavy dynamic exercise.[98,101]

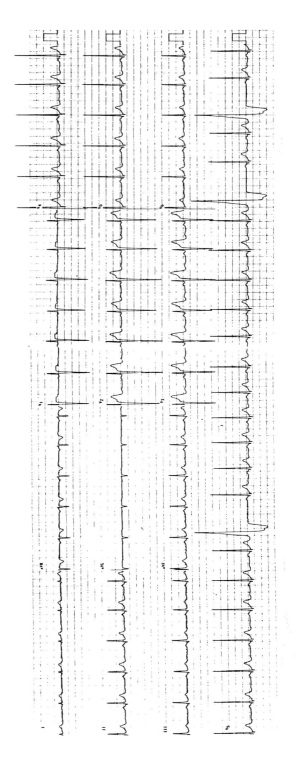

Figure 4. Early repolarization (ST segment and J point elevation), prominent U-waves and high voltages in the electrocardiogram of an 18-year old male tennis-player.

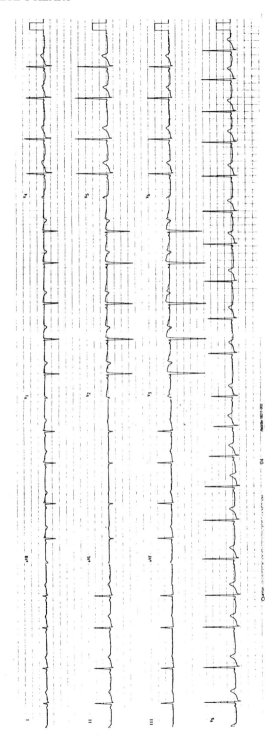

Figure 5. J point depression and asymmetric negative T waves in leads V1 to V3 in the electrocardiograms of a 19-year old female tennis player. Echocardiographic examination revealed no abnormalities.

Regression of left ventricular hypertrophy

It has been shown in several longitudinal studies that deconditioning of athletes results in regression of training-induced cardiac hypertrophy.[102-105] Most studies have shown regression of training-induced left ventricular hypertrophy to occur in several (3-12) weeks, characterized by considerable (15-30%) reduction of left ventricular wall thickness and diameter.[102-107] Saltin et al.[108] demonstrated a decrease of 11.9% in heart size in 5 athletes after three weeks of bed rest (Figure 6). Maron et al.[104] measured a 24% reduction of left ventricular mass and of left ventricular wall thickness in 6 Olympic athletes after 13 weeks of deconditioning. Two other studies demonstrated 20% and 40% decreases in left ventricular mass after only 3 weeks of inactivity.[106,107] It is therefore clear that discontinuation of training may lead to rapid reversal of training-induced cardiac enlargement and left ventricular hypertrophy in healthy young subjects.

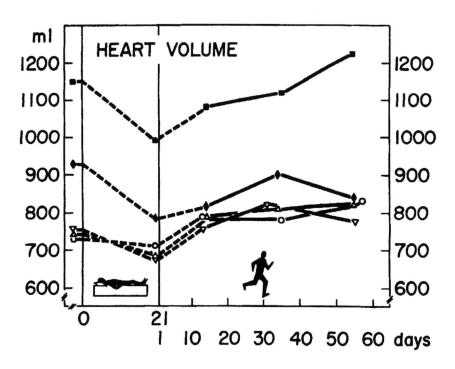

Figure 6. Changes in radiographic heart volume after 3 weeks of 24 hour bed rest. Individual data of 5 subjects before and after bed rest and at different intervals during training. From Saltin et al. Circulation 1968, 38:1-78. Reprinted with permission.[108]

However, the question remains whether life-long intense competitive training may lead to delayed damage and transition to pathological forms of hypertrophy. In the study by Höglund et al.,[51] left ventricular dimensions and mass of former athletes were normal compared to sedentary control subjects, although the left atrial dimension remained enlarged. Dickhuth et al.[104] re-examined 38 world-class athletes, for whom results of an exercise ECG and radiological heart volume measurements were available from their active competitive period, 24 years after their initial examination. They observed that former athletes, who were now totally inactive, showed left ventricular mass and size in the upper normal range, with a maximum oxygen capacity clearly exceeding the norm. The former athletes who were still active had significantly increased left ventricular mass and size, suggesting that normalization of left ventricular hypertrophy depends only partly on the actual physical activity. In the study by Vollmer-Larsen et al.,[110] no significant difference in cardiac structure and function was found between former athletes and the control group. Fardy et al.[111] found slightly increased myocardial function parameters in 350 former athletes compared with 156 non-athletes. It has been suggested that in former athletes who have participated in strenuous training for a very long period of time the cardiac hypertrophy may be partly irreversible.[64,65,112] However, the majority of the studies indicate that exercise-induced left ventricular hypertrophy is completely reversible, without development of pathological hypertrophy.

When athletes suddenly retire from active competitive sports, some athletes temporarily suffer from arrhythmias and palpitations. This has been explained by Pavlik et al.[113] as a result of persisting cardiac enlargement and bradycardia associated with a temporarily unstable autonomous control, with high sympathetic and parasympathetic drive. This may lead to a hyperkinesis-like syndrome with an increased cardiac output. To prevent this phenomenon, retiring from highly competitive sports should be done gradually.

Conclusions

The "athlete's heart" is characterized by bradycardia at rest, an increased left ventricular stroke volume, increased left ventricular cavity size and wall thickness, an increased left ventricular mass, brady-arrhythmias, and well-defined electrocardiographic criteria for left ventricular hypertrophy. Common brady-arrhythmias in the athlete's heart include sinus

References

1. Maron BJ. Structural features of the athlete heart as defined by echocardiography. J Am Coll Cardiol 1986;7:190-203.
2. Keul J, Dickhuth HH, Lehmann M, Staiger J. The athlete's heart- haemodynamics and structure. Int J Sports Med 1982;3:33-43.
3. Björnstad H, Storstein L, Meen HD, Hals O. Electrocardiographic findings of repolarization in athletic students and control subjects. Cardiology 1994;84:51-60.
4   Huston TP, Puffer JC, Rodney WM. The athletic heart syndrome. N Engl J Med 1985;313:24-31.
5. Osler W. The principles and practice of medicine. New York, D. Appleton; 1892: p 635.
6. Henschen SE. Uppsala universitets Årsskrift 1897. Uppsala: Akademiska bokhandeln; 1898: p 14.
7. Moritz F. Größe und Form des Herzens bei Meistern im Sport. Dtsch Arch Klin Med 1934;176:455-66.
8. Lysholm E, Nylin G, Quarnå K. The relation between the heart volume and stroke volume under physiological and pathological conditions. Acta Radiol 1934;15:237-57.
9. Deutsch F, Kauf E. Herz und Sport. Berlin: Urban & Schwarzenberg; 1924.
10. Kaufmann W. Die Beeinflußung der Herzgröße durch Arbeit und Sport. Med Welt 1933;7:1347-8.
11. Friedberg C. Erkrankungen des Herzens. Stuttgart: Thieme Verlag; 1972.
12. Wesslén L, Påhlson C, Lindquist O, et al. An increase in sudden unexpected cardiac deaths among young Swedish orienteers during 1979-1992. Eur Heart J 1996;17:902-10.
13. Carrière EGJ. Plotse dood bij topsport. Utrecht: Rijksuniversiteit; 1992.
14. Keren G, Shoenfeld Y. Sudden death and physical exertion. J Sports Cardiol 1981;21:90-3.
15. Oakley DG, Oakley CM. Significance of abnormal electrocardiograms in highly trained athletes. Am J Cardiol 1982;50:985-9.
16. Levy D, Garrison RJ, Savage DD, Kannel WB, Castelli WP. Prognostic implications of echocardiographically determined left ventricular mass in the Framingham Heart Study. N Engl J Med 1990;322:1561-6.
17. Reindell H, Musshoff K, Klepzig H. Die physiologische und krankhafte Hervergrösserung. In: Klepzig H, editors. Die Funktionsdiagnostik des Herzens. Berlin: Springer-Verlag; 1958: p. 128-44.
18. Lichtman J, O'Rourke RA, Klein A, Karliner JS. Electrocardiogram of the athlete: alterations simulating those of organic heart disease. Arch Intern Med 1973;132:763-70.
19. Kjellberg SR, Rudhe U, Sjöstrand T. The relation of the cardiac volume to the weight and surface area of the body, the blood volume and the physical capacity for work. Acta Radiol 1949;31:113-22.
20. Sokolow M, Lyon TP. The ventricular complex in left ventricular hypertrophy as obtained by unipolar precordial and limb leads. Am Heart J 1949;37:161-86.

21. Sokolow M, Lyon TP. Ventricular complex in right ventricular hypertrophy as obtained by unipolar precordial and limb leads. Am Heart J 1949;38:273-94.
22. Kirch E. Anatomische Grundlagen des Sportherzens. Verh Dtsch Ges Inn Med 1935;47:73-98.
23. Kirch E. Herzkräftigung und echte Herzhypertrophie durch Sport. Z Kreislaufforsch 1936;28:893-907.
24. Linzbach AJ. Struktur und Funktion des gesunden und kranken Herzens. In: Klepzig H, editor. Die Funktionsdiagnostik des Herzens. Berlin: Springer-Verlag; 1958. p. 94-115.
25. Dickhuth HH, Jakob E, Wink K, Bonzel T, Keul J, Just H. Läßt sich aus der maximalen physiologischen Herzhypertrophie ein absolutes kritisches Herzgewicht ableiten? In: Franz I, Mellerowicz H, Noack W, editors. Training und Sport zur Prävention und Rehabilitation in der technisierten Umwelt. Berlin: Springer-Verlag; 1985, p. 722-7.
26. Messerli FH. Pathophysiology of left ventricular hypertrophy. In: Messerli F, editors. Left ventricular hypertrophy and its regression. London: Science Press; 1996. p. 2.1-2.15.
27. Levy D, Garrison RJ, Savage DD, Kannel WB, Castelli WP. Left ventricular mass and incidence of coronary heart disease in an elderly cohort: the Framingham Heart Study. Ann Intern Med 1989;110:101-7.
28. Talan DA, Bauernfeind RA, Ashley WW, Kanakis C, Rosen KM. Twenty-four hour continuous ECG recordings in long-distance runners. Chest 1982;82:19-24.
29. Viitasalo MT, Kala R, Eisalo A. Ambulatory electrocardiographic recording in endurance athletes. Br Heart J 1982;47:213-20.
30. Northcote RJ, MacFarlane P, Ballantyne D. Ambulatory electrocardiography in squash players. Br Heart J 1983;50:372-7.
31. Palatini P, Maraglino G, Sperti G, et al. Prevalence and possible mechanisms of ventricular arrhythmias in athletes. Am Heart J 1985;110:560-7.
32. Kennedy HL, Whitlock JA, Sprague MK, Kennedy LJ, Buckingham TA, Goldberg RJ. Long-term

follow-up of asymptomatic healthy subjects with frequent and complex ventricular ectopy. N Engl J Med 1985;312:193-7.

33.   Kujala UM, Sarna S, Kaprio J, Koskenvuo M. Hospital care in later life among former world-class Finnish athletes. JAMA 1996;276:216-20.

34.   Sarna S, Sahi T, Koskenvuo M, Kaprio J. Increased life expectancy of world class male athletes. Med Sci Sports Exerc 1993;25:237-44.

35.   Lee IM, Hsieh CC, Paffenberger RS. Exercise intensity and longevity in men. JAMA 1995;273:1179-84.

36.   Siscovick DS, Weiss NS, Fletcher RH, Lasky T. The incidence of primary cardiac arrest during vigorous exercise. N Engl J Med 1984;311:874-7.

37.   Blair SN, Kampert JB, Kohl III HW, et al. Influences of cardiorespiratory fitness and other precursors on cardiovascular disease and all-cause mortality in men and women. JAMA 1996;276:205-10.

38.   Lakka TA, Venäläinen JM, Rauramaa R, Salonen R, Tuomilehto J, Salonen JT. Relation of leisure-time physical activity and cardiorespiratory fitness to the risk of acute myocardial infarction in men. N Engl J Med 1994;330:1549-54.

39.   Berlin JA, Colditz GA. A meta-analysis of physical activity in the prevention of coronary heart disease. Am J Epidemiol 1990;132:612-28.

40.   Winget JF, Capeless MA, Ades PA. Sudden death in athletes. Sports Med 1994;18:375-83.

41.   Maron BJ, Shirani J, Poliac LC, Mathenge R, Roberts WC, Mueller FO. Sudden death in young competitive athletes. JAMA 1996;276:199-204.

42.   Zeppilli P, Santini C, Palmieri V, Vannicelli R, Giordano A, Frustaci A. Role of myocarditis in athletes with minor arrhythmias and/or echocardiographic abnormalities. Chest 1994;106:373-80.

43.   Virmani R, Burke AP, Farb A, Kark JA. Causes of sudden death in young and middle-aged competitive athletes. Cardiol Clin 1997;15:439-66.

44.   Epstein SE, Maron BJ. Sudden death and the competitive athlete: perspectives on preparticipation studies. J Am Coll Cardiol 1986;7:220-30.

45.   Phillips M, Robinowitz M, Higgins JR, Boran KJ, Reed T, Virmani R. Sudden cardiac death in air force recruits. JAMA 1986;256:2696-9.

46.   Grossman W, Jones D, McLaurin LP. Wall stress and patterns of hypertrophy in the human left ventricle. J Clin Invest 1975;56:56-64.

47.   Swynghedauw B. Molecular cardiology for the cardiologist. Dordrecht: Kluwer Academic Publishers; 1995. p. 120.

48.   Stratton JR, Levy WC, Cerqueira MD, Schwartz RS, Abrass IB. Cardiovascular responses to exercise. Circulation 1994;89:1648-55.

49.   Pellicia A, Maron BJ, Spataro A, Proschan MA, Spirito P. The upper limit of physiological cardiac hypertrophy in highly trained elite athletes. N Engl J Med 1991;324:295-301.

50.   Hauser AM, Dressendorfer RH, Vos M, Hashimoto T, Gordon S, Timmis GC. Symmetric cardiac enlargement in highly trained endurance athletes: a two-dimensional echocardiographic study. Am Heart J 1985;109:1038-44.

51.   Höglund C. Enlarged left atrial dimension in former endurance athletes: an echocardiographic study. Int J Sports Med 1986;7:133-6.

52.   Mumford M, Prakash R. Electrocardiographic and echocardiographic characteristics of long distance runners. Am J Sports Med 1981;9:23-8.

53.   Roeske WR, O'Rourke RA, Klein A, Leopold G, Karliner JS. Noninvasive evaluation of ventricular hypertrophy in professional athletes. Circulation 1976;53:286-91.

54.   Pellicia A. Determinants of morphologic cardiac adaptation in elite athletes: the role of athletic training and constitutional factors. Int J Sports Med 1996;17:157-63.

55.   Urhausen A, Monz T, Kindermann W. Sports-specific adaptation of left ventricular muscle mass in athlete's heart. I. An echocardiographic study with combined isometric and dynamic exercise trained athletes (male and female rowers). Int J Sports Med 1996;17:145-51.

56.   Urhausen A, Monz T, Kindermann W. Sports-specific adaptation of left ventricular mass in athlete's heart. II. An echocardiographic study with 400-m runners and soccer players. Int J Sports Med 1996;17:152-6.

57.   Morganroth J, Maron BJ, Henry WL, Epstein SE. Comparative left ventricular dimensions in trained athletes. Ann Intern Med 1975;82:521-4.

58.   MacDougall JD, Tuxen D, Sale DG, Moroz JR, Sutton JR. Arterial blood pressure response to heavy resistance exercise. Am J Physiol 1985;58:785-90.

59.   Clifford PS, Hanel B, Secher NH. Arterial blood pressure response to rowing. Med Sci Sports Exerc 1994;26:715-9.

60.   Pellicia A, Maron BJ, Culasso F, Spataro A, Caselli G. Athlete's heart in women: echocardiographic characterization of highly trained elite female athletes. JAMA 1996;276:211-5.

61.   Milliken MC, Stray-Gundersen J, Peshock RM, Katz J, Mitchell JH. Left ventricular mass as determined by

magnetic resonance imaging in male endurance athletes. Am J Cardiol 1988;62:301-5.

62. Fleck SJ, Henke C, Wilson W. Cardiac MRI of elite junior Olympic weight lifters. Int J Sports Med 1989;10:329-33.

63. Riley-Hagan M, Peshock RM, Stray-Gundersen J, Katz J, Ryschon TW, Mitchell JH. Left ventricular dimensions and mass using magnetic resonance imaging in female endurance athletes. Am J Cardiol 1992;69:1067-74.

64. Pluim BM, Chin JC, De Roos A, et al. Cardiac anatomy, function and metablosim in elite cyclists assessed by magnetic resonance imaging and spectroscopy. Eur Heart J 1996;17:1271-8.

65. Pluim BM, Lamb HJ, Kayser HWM, et al. Functional and metabolic evaluation of the athlete's heart by magnetic resonance imaging and dobutamine stress magnetic resonance spectroscopy. Circulation 1998;97:666-72.

66. Nishimura T, Yamada Y, Kawai C. Echocardiographic evaluation of long-term effects of exercise on left ventricular hypertrophy and function in professional bicyclists. Circulation 1980;61:832-40.

67. Miki T, Yokota Y, Seo T, Yokoyama M. Echocardiographic findings in 104 professional cyclists with follow-up study. Am Heart J 1994;127:898-905.

68. Little WC, Downes TR. Clinical evaluation of left ventricular diastolic performance. Prog Cardiovasc Dis 1990;32:273-90.

69. Zile MR. Diastolic dysfunction: detection, consequences, and treatment. Part 2: diagnosis and treatment of diastolic dysfunction. Mod Concepts Cardiovasc Dis 1990;59:1-6.

70. Inouye I, Massie B, Loge BS, et al. Abnormal left ventricular filling: an early finding in mild to moderate systemic hypertension. Am J Cardiol 1984;53:120-6.

71. Smith VE, Schulman P, Karimeddini MK, White WB, Meeran MK, Katz AM. Rapid ventricular filling in left ventricular hypertrophy: II. Pathologic hypertrophy. J Am Coll Cardiol 1985;5:869-74.

72. Nixon JV, Wright AR, Porter TR, Roy V, Arrowood JA. Effects of exercise on left ventricular diastolic performance in trained athletes. Am J Cardiol 1991;68:945-9.

73. Granger CB, Karimeddini MK, Smith V-E, Shapiro HR, Katz AM, Riba AL. Rapid ventricular filling in left ventricular hypertrophy: 1. Physiologic hypertrophy. J Am Coll Cardiol 1985;5:862-8.

74. Matsuda M, Sugishita Y, Koseki S, Ito I, Akatsuka T, Takamatsu K. Effect of exercise on left ventricular diastolic filling in athletes and nonathletes. J Appl Physiol 1983;55:323-8.

75. Galanti G, Comeglio M, Vinci M, Cappelli B, Vono MC, Bamoshmoosh M. Echocardiographic Doppler evaluation of left ventricular diastolic function in athletes' hypertrophied hearts. J Vasc Dis 1993;44:341-6.

76. Forman DE, Manning WJ, Hauser R, Gervino EV, Evans WJ, Wei JY. Enhanced left ventricular diastolic filling associated with long-term endurance training. J Gerontol 1992;47:56-8.

77. Douglas PS, O'Toole ML, Hiller WD, Hackney K, Reichek N. Cardiac fatigue after prolonged exercise. Circulation 1987;76:1206-13.

78. Braunwald E, Kloner RA. The stunned myocardium: prolonged, postischemic ventricular dysfunction. Circulation 1982;66:1146-9.

79. Starnes JW, Bowles DK. Role of exercise in the cause and prevention of cardiac dysfunction. Exerc Sport Sci Rev 1995;23:349-73.

80. Vanoverschelde JJ, LT Younis, JA Melin, et al. Prolonged exercise induces left ventricular dysfunction in healthy subjects. J Appl Physiol 1991;70:1356-63.

81. Israel S. Die Herzfunktion bei trainingsbedingten extremen Bradykardien von 29...34 min[-1]. Med Sport 1975;7:197-202.

82. Ekblom B, Kilbom A, Soltysiak J. Physical training, bradycardia, and autonomic nervous system. Scand J Clin Lab Invest 1973;32:251-6.

83. Kenney WL. Parasympathetic control of resting heart rate: relationship to aerobic power. Med Sci Sports Exerc 1985;17:451-5.

84. Smith ML, Hudson DL, Graitzer HM, Raven PB. Exercise training bradycardia: the role of autonomic balance. Med Sci Sports Exerc 1989;21:40-4.

85. Zehender M, Meinertz T, Keul J, Just H. ECG variants and cardiac arrhythmias in athletes: clinical relevance and prognostic importance. Am Heart J 1990;119:1378-91.

86. Schamroth L, Jokl E. Marked sinus and A-V nodal bradycardia with interference-dissociation in an athlete. J Sports Med 1969;9:128-9.

87. Rost R, Hollman W. Athlete's heart - a review of its historical assessment and new aspects. Int J Sports Med 1983;4:147-65.

88. Carre F, Chignon JC. Advantages of electrocardiographic monitoring in top level athletes. Int J Sports Med 1991;12:236-40.

89. Viitasalo MT, Kala R, Eisalo A. Ambulatory electrocardiographic findings in young athletes between 14 and 16 years of age. Eur Heart J 1984;5:2-6.

90. Rowland TW, Delaney BC, Siconolfi SF. 'Athlete's heart' in prepubertal children. Pediatrics 1987;79:800-4.

91. Pokan R, Huonker M, Schumacher M, et al. Das EKG des Sportherzens. Acta Med Aust 1994;21:76-82.
92. Douglas PS, O'Toole ML, Hiller WDB, Hackney K, Reichek N. Electrocardiographic diagnosis of exercise-induced left ventricular hypertrophy. Am Heart J 1988;116:784-90.
93. Pantano JA, Oriel RJ. Prevalence and nature of cardiac arrhythmias in apparently normal well-trained runners. Am Heart J 1982;104:762-8.
94. Pilcher GF, Cook J, Johnston BL, Fletcher GF. Twenty-four-hour continuous electrocardiography during exercise and free activity in 80 apparently healthy runners. Am J Cardiol 1983;52:859-61.
95. Hanne-Paparo N, Drory Y, Schoenfeld Y, Shapiro Y, Kellerman JJ. Common ECG changes in athletes. Cardiology 1976;61:267-78.
96. Zeppilli P, Pirrami MM, Sassara M, Fenici R. Ventricular repolarization disturbances in athlete: standardization of terminology, ethiopathogenetic spectrum and pathophysiological mechanisms. J Sports Cardiol 1981;21:322-35.
97. Task Force of the European Society of Cardiology and the North American Society of Pacing and Electrophysiology. Heart rate variability. Circulation 1996;93:1043-65.
98. Seals DR, Chase PB. Influence of physical training on heart rate variability and baroreflex circulatory control. J Appl Physiol 1989;66:1886-95.
99. Goldsmith RL, Bigger T, Steinman RC, Fleiss JL. Comparison of 24-hour parasympathetic activity in endurance-trained and untrained young men. J Am Coll Cardiol 1992;20:552-8.
100. Reiling MJ, Seals DR. Respiratory sinus arrhythmia and carotid baroreflex control of heart rate in endurance athletes and untrained controls. Clin Physiol 1988;8:511-9.
101. Furlan R, Piazza S, Dell'Orto S, Gentile E, Cerutti S, Pagani M, Malliani A. Early and late effects of exercise and athletic training on neural mechanisms controlling heart rate. Cardiovasc Res 1993;27:482-8.
102. Dickhuth HH, Reindell H, Lehmann M, Keul J. Ruckbildungsfähigkeit des Sportherzens. Z Kardiol 1985;74:135-43.
103. Fagard R, Aubert A, Lysens R, Staessen J, Vanhees L, Amery A. Noninvasive assessment of seasonal variations in cardiac structure and function in cyclists. Circulation 1983;67:896-900.
104. Maron BJ, Pellicia A, Spataro A, Granata M. Reduction in left ventricular wall thickness after deconditioning in highly trained Olympic athletes. Br Heart J 1993;69:125-8.
105. Ehsani AA, Hagberg JM, Hickson RC. Rapid changes in left ventricular dimensions and mass in response to physical conditioning and deconditioning. Am J Cardiol 1978;42:52-6.
106. Martin WD[3rd], Coyle EF, Bloomfield SA, Ehsani AA. Effects of physical deconditioning after intense endurance training on left ventricular dimensions and stroke volume. J Am Coll Cardiol 1986;7:982-9.
107. Ehsani AA. Loss of cardiovascular adaptations after cessation of training. Cardiol Clin 1992;2:257-66.
108. Saltin B, Blomqvist G, Mitchell JH, Johnson RL Jr, Wildenthal K, Chapman CB. Response to exercise after bed rest and training. Circulation 1968;38(5 Suppl):VII1-78.
109. Dickhuth HH, Hortsmann T, Staiger J, Reindell H, Keul J. The long-term involution of physiological cardiomegaly and cardiac hypertrophy. Med Sci Sports Exerc 1989;21:244-9.
110. Vollmer-Larsen A, Vollmer-Larsen B, Kelbaek H, Godtfredsen J. The veteran athlete: an echocardiographic comparison of veteran cyclists, former cyclists and non-athletic subjects. Acta Physiol Scand 1989;135:393-8.
111. Hardy PS, Maresh CM, Abbott RD. A comparison of myocardial function in former athletes and non-athletes. Med Sci Sports Exerc 1976;8:26-30.
112. Roskamm H, Reindel H, Weissleder H, Kessler G, Aletter K. Zur Frage der Spätschäden nach intensivem Hochleistungssport. Med Welt 1964;41:2170-80.
113. Pavlik G, Bachl N, Wollein W, Làngfy Gy, Prokop L. Resting echocardiographic parameters after cessation of regular endurance training. Int J Sports Med 1986;7:226-31.

8. LEFT VENTRICULAR HYPERTROPHIC HEART DISEASE STUDIED BY MR IMAGING AND ^{31}P-MR SPECTROSCOPY

H.J. LAMB, A. DE ROOS, E.E. VAN DER WALL

Summary

Left ventricular hypertrophy (LVH) can be associated with systolic and/or diastolic function abnormalities as well as with changes in high-energy phosphate (HEP) metabolism. The current chapter aims to provide an overview of clinically applicable techniques for MR imaging and phosphorus-31 (^{31}P)-MR spectroscopy to study the human left ventricle. The hypertensive heart, athlete's heart and hypertrophied heart due to aortic valve stenosis/regurgitation are compared with regard to changes in LV function and HEP metabolism. It is shown that diastolic LV function and myocardial HEP metabolism are impaired only when LVH is caused by permanent pressure or volume overload, and not by a temporary increase in cardiac workload during part of the day as in elite athletes. In addition, there is an association between impaired LV diastolic function and altered myocardial HEP metabolism in patients with hypertension and in patients with aortic valve disease.

Introduction

LVH is a recognised risk factor for cardiac morbidity and mortality.[1] LVH is most likely caused by *permanent* cardiovascular overload which causes myocyte stretch and increased angiotensin II concentrations in vascular and myocardial tissue[2] which is believed to trigger "genetic reprogramming".[3] This process promotes cell growth and extracellular matrix production, leading to an increase in myocardial mass and increased LV stiffness. Continuous cardiac overload can be caused by pathologic conditions, such as the presence of systemic hypertension or aortic valve disease. On the other hand, supernormal physical

E. E. van der Wall et al.(eds.), Left Ventricular Hypertrophy, 107-119.
© 1999 *Kluwer Academic Publishers. Printed in the Netherlands.*

exercise, as in elite athletes, increases cardiac workload during part of the day. In all previously mentioned groups LVH is a common observation.

LVH can be associated with systolic and/or diastolic dysfunction.[4,5] Previous animal studies have revealed that LVH can also be accompanied by alterations in the myocardial HEP metabolism.[6,7] Magnetic resonance (MR) imaging is a highly reliable technique for assessment of LV dimensions and systolic and diastolic function.[8,9] ^{31}P-MR spectroscopy is a noninvasive reproducible method to study myocardial HEP metabolism *in vivo*.[10-12] The combination of functional and metabolic evaluation of the human heart in a single MR examination may ultimately provide a sensitive tool for early detection of changes in cardiac performance and myocardial viability.

In this chapter, an overview will be given of the functional and metabolic consequences of LV overload in patients with hypertension, in patients with aortic valve disease, and in elite athletes. The feasibility of MR imaging and ^{31}P-MR spectroscopy will be discussed to evaluate LV systolic and diastolic function and myocardial HEP metabolism. Comparison of the functional and metabolic state of the human heart with LVH of different origin may provide new (patho)physiological insights.

Magnetic resonance imaging

MR imaging using gradient-echo techniques provides an excellent tool for evaluating cardiac function.[13-15] MR images have good contrast between the blood pool and myocardium and reveal cardiac flow and function dynamically using the movie-loop display. An imaging protocol[16] to acquire basic functional LV parameters is described here; based on images in the transverse plane (Figure 1) right anterior oblique equivalent (two-chamber view) images are centered through the apex of the LV to intersect the mitral valve plane. To acquire a four-chamber view a slice is positioned to transect the apex of the LV on the diastolic and systolic two-chamber images and is centered low on the mitral valve plane (Figure 1). Planned on the diastolic and systolic two-chamber and four-chamber images, the heart is imaged from apex to base with 10 imaging levels in the short-axis orientation (Figure 2).

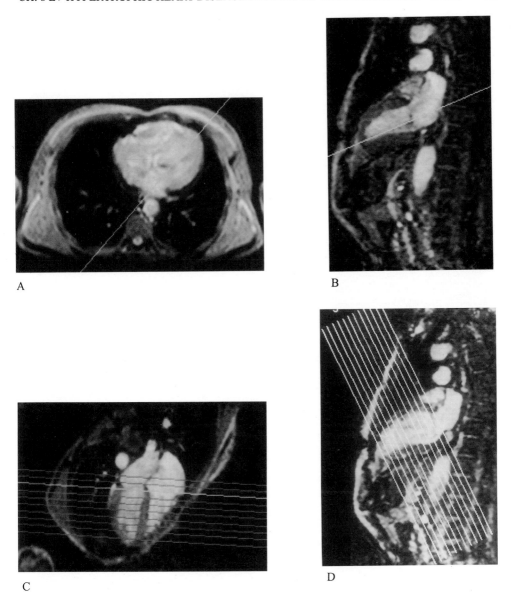

Figure 1. (A) Transverse survey image at the level of the mitral valve obtained with segmented echo-planar MR imaging (EPI) during a 10s breath-hold. The two-chamber view is obtained by positioning the center of a slice in the middle of the mitral valve on this image and thereafter by angulating the slice through the apex in the lowest transverse survey image to show blood signal (not shown). (B) Two-chamber view in the end-systolic time frame, acquired with multishot EPI during a 10s breath-hold. During this acquisition time 23 images were obtained to provide a cine movie-loop of the cardiac contraction. On this image and the accompanying end-diastolic image (not shown) the four-chamber view was planned. The slice center was positioned just below the center of the mitral valve in the end-systolic image and angulated through the apex. (C) Four chamber view at end-systole, acquired with segmented EPI during a 10s breath-hold. From the end-diastolic (not shown) and end-systolic images in the two-chamber view (D) and four-chamber view (C) the short-axis scan is planned. Slices were positioned perpendicular to the long-axis of the LV, which is from the midmitral point to the apex. The resulting stack of short-axis views is shown in Figure 2.

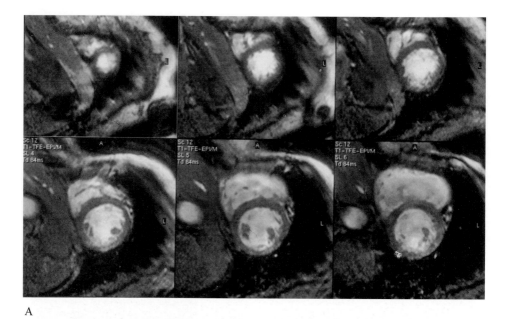

A

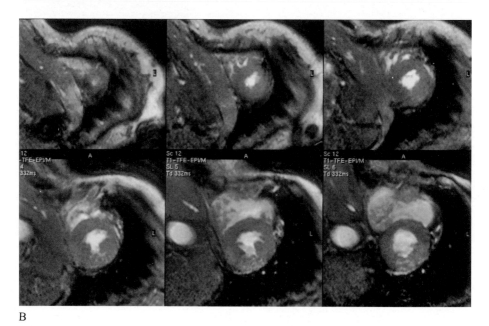

B

Figure 2. Short-axis views of the LV of a healthy volunteer acquired with multishot EPI at end-diastole (A) and end-systole (B). Six slices are shown out of a dataset covering the entire LV. For review of the scan setup, see text and Figure 1.

A previous study[16] showed that double-oblique, fast evaluation of LV mass and systolic and diastolic function is possible using a multishot echo-planar MR imaging (EPI) technique with breath-holding, with superior image quality as compared to conventional gradient echo MR imaging (Figure 3). EPI allows acquisition of MR images covering the entire heart in about 7 minutes, whereas conventional gradient echo imaging requires 45 minutes to obtain the same image set. EPI-derived measurements are at least as accurate as data obtained from conventional MR imaging.[16] Absence of respiratory artefacts contributes to more reproducible and faster detection of endocardial and epicardial borders of the LV, thereby improving functional evaluation of the heart.

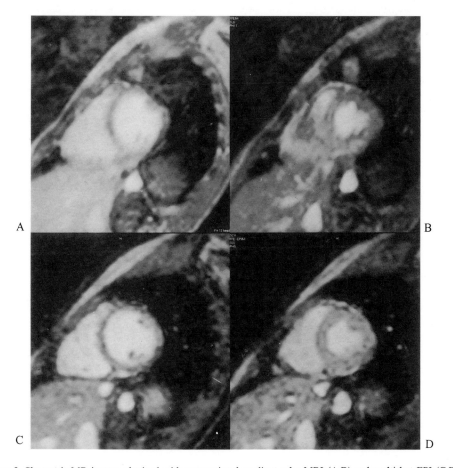

Figure 3. Short-axis MR images obtained with conventional gradient echo MRI (A,B) and multishot EPI (C,D) are shown at end-diastole (A, C) and end-systole (B, D).[16] Note the typical breathing artefacts on the diastolic gradient echo image (A), such as signal voids in the anterolateral region of the LV and the fuzzy epicardial border at the posterior wall. Note differences in edge sharpness and contrast between blood and myocardium.

Phosphorus magnetic resonance spectroscopy

Phosphorus-31 magnetic resonance (^{31}P-MR) spectroscopy is a unique, noninvasive tool to study high-energy phosphate (HEP) metabolism of the human heart *in vivo*.[10-12] Hence ^{31}P-MR spectroscopy may disclose metabolic derangements associated with underlying heart disease, such as myocardial ischemia, cardiomyopathy and hypertrophy.[17-19] Several important metabolic parameters can be extracted from the spectroscopic data, such as intracellular myocardial pH, levels of inorganic phosphate (P_i), phosphocreatine (PCr), adenosine-triphosphate (ATP) and their ratios PCr/P_i, P_i/ATP and PCr/ATP.[20] At an external magnetic field of 1.5-T, the ^{31}P-MR signal of P_i in the normal heart is small and difficult to resolve from overlapping blood signal, even when applying proton decoupling.[18] Therefore, the PCr/ATP ratio is the most commonly used spectroscopic parameter in human cardiac ^{31}P-MR spectroscopy studies. Figure 4 shows an example of a typical ^{31}P-MR spectrum with resonance peak assignments.

Hypertensive and athlete's heart

To evaluate LV function and HEP metabolism in patients with hypertensive heart disease, eleven male patients with hypertension[21] and thirteen matched healthy subjects were studied.[22] In addition, 21 elite male cyclists with normal blood pressures and 12 matched healthy controls were studied.[23] Both groups of study subjects were submitted to MR imaging at rest[16] and ^{31}P-MRS at rest and during high-dose atropine-dobutamine (A-D) stress[24] Figure 5 shows the hemodynamic response to the stress test.

Hypertensive patients showed higher LV mass (98 ± 28 g/m^2) than healthy controls (73 ± 13 g/m^2, p<0.01). LV filling was impaired in patients, reflected by a decreased peak rate of wall thinning (PRWThn), E/A ratio, early peak filling rate, and early deceleration peak (all p<0.05), whereas systolic function was still normal. Figure 6 and 7 respectively show individual ^{31}P-MR spectra and an overview of all spectroscopic data. The myocardial PCr/ATP ratio determined in patients at rest (1.20 ± 0.18) and during stress (0.95 ± 0.25) was lower than corresponding values obtained from healthy controls at rest (1.39 ± 0.17, p<0.05) and during stress (1.16 ± 0.18, *P*<0.05). The PCr/ATP ratio correlated significantly with

PRWThn (r= –0.55, P<0.01) and early deceleration peak (r= –0.56, P<0.01). Myocardial PCr/ATP did not correlate to LV mass index.

Elite cyclists showed higher LV mass (102±10 g/m^2) than healthy controls (69±6 g/m^2, P<0.001). There were no statistically significant differences between cyclists and control subjects regarding LV ejection fraction, cardiac index, early (E) and atrial (A) peak filling rate, E/A ratio, and early deceleration peak (all p>0.05). Myocardial PCr/ATP determined at rest in cyclists (1.41±0.20) and controls (1.41±0.18) was similar and decreased to the same extent during stress in athletes (1.16±0.13) and healthy subjects (1.21±0.20). The decrease due to A-D stress was highly significant in both groups (p<0.001). Myocardial PCr/ATP did not correlate to LV mass index or measures of LV function.

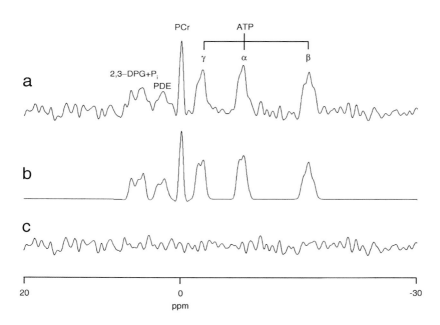

Figure 4. Cardiac ^{31}P-MR spectrum of the left ventricle of a healthy volunteer at rest obtained with three-dimensional volume selection using ISIS. The acquired spectrum (a) shows resonance peaks of phosphocreatine (PCr), adenosine-triphosphate (ATP), phosphodiesters (PDE) like blood phospholipids and glycerophosphorylcholine, and the combined signal of 2,3-diphosphoglycerate (2,3-DPG) originating from blood and inorganic phosphate (P$_i$). A PCr/ATP ratio of 1.00±0.10 (10%) was derived from the simulated spectrum (b). The difference between acquired and simulated spectra (c) shows no residual signals and illustrates a low spectral noise level. The rCRSD of 10% corresponded to a SNR of 9.7 measured from the acquired spectrum (a). The model fitting was performed automatically in the time domain. Exponential line broadening of 15 Hz was applied.

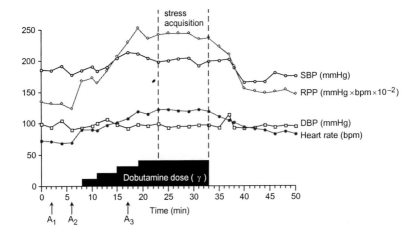

Figure 5. Example of hemodynamic changes due to A-D stress in a 55-year-old male patient with hypertensive heart disease. Atropine sulfate was administered in three doses (A_1 to A_3), the dobutamine infusion rate (microg/kg/min) is indicated by the dark area. ^{31}P-MR spectra acquired at rest and during A-D stress from this patient are shown in Figure 6. Abbreviations: SBP, systolic blood pressure (mmHg); DBP, diastolic blood pressure (mmHg); bpm, beats per min; RPP, rate-pressure product (mmHg×bpm×10^{-2}).

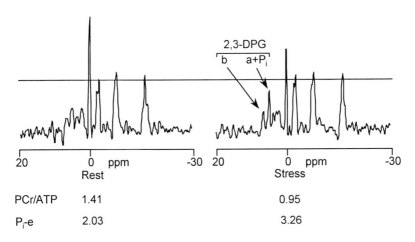

	Rest	Stress
PCr/ATP	1.41	0.95
P_i-e	2.03	3.26

Figure 6. ^{31}P-MR spectra obtained at rest and during A-D stress from the anterior wall of the LV of a patient with hypertensive heart disease. Hemodynamic changes due to A-D infusion in this particular patient are shown in Figure 5. Values of myocardial PCr/ATP and P_i-e are presented below the ^{31}P-MR spectra. Myocardial PCr/ATP ratios were corrected for partial saturation effects and blood-ATP contamination, and line broadening of 15 Hz was applied. The inorganic phosphate (P_i) signal is obscured by overlapping signal from 2,3-diphosphoglycerate (2,3-DPG), which consists of two separate resonance peaks. When the 2,3-DPG_a+P_i peak increases while the 2,3-DPG_b peak is unchanged, the change in signal is most likely caused by an increase in P_i. Therefore, a semiquantitative estimate of P_i signal intensity (P_i-e) was obtained by the ratio: (DPG_a+P_i)/DPG_b, a dimensionless parameter.

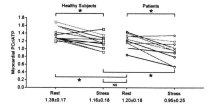
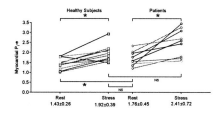

Figure 7. Changes in myocardial PCr/ATP (left) and myocardial P_i-e (right) due to severe A-D-induced stress in healthy subjects and patients with hypertensive heart disease. Note the transient decrease in myocardial PCr/ATP and increase in P_i-e from rest in healthy subjects, rest in patients, stress in healthy subjects to stress in patients. Average values for myocardial PCr/ATP and P_i-e at rest and during stress are given below the Figure (mean ± SD). * P<0.05; NS, not statistically significant (p>0.05).

Aortic valve disease

MR imaging at rest was performed shortly before aortic valve replacement in 27 male patients with severe aortic valve disease (19 aortic stenosis, 8 aortic regurgitation). The control group consisted of 10 matched healthy volunteers who underwent both MR imaging and ^{31}P-MR spectroscopy at rest[11] From the 27 patients, a subgroup of 18 patients (14 aortic stenosis, 4 aortic regurgitation) also underwent ^{31}P-MRS at rest.[11] Obviously, A-D stress testing could not be performed in these patients with aortic valve disease for safety reasons.

LV mass was increased in patients with aortic stenosis (131 ± 30 g/m^2), and in patients with aortic regurgitation (150 ± 34 g/m^2), as compared to LV mass of the matched healthy controls (69 ± 6 g/m^2, all p<0.05). Figure 8 shows examples of MR images in a patient with aortic valve stenosis combined with mitral valve regurgitation. Diastolic function was impaired in both subgroups of patients with aortic valve disease, whereas systolic function was still normal as compared to the healthy subjects. Myocardial PCr/ATP ratio determined at rest in the subgroup of 18 patients with aortic valve disease (1.24 ± 0.17) was lower than values obtained from healthy controls at rest (1.43 ± 0.14, p<0.01). Myocardial PCr/ATP acquired in patients with aortic stenosis (1.28 ± 0.16) was similar to values obtained in patients with aortic regurgitation (1.11 ± 0.22, p>0.05). Myocardial PCr/ATP correlated significantly with the early deceleration peak (r= −0.39, p<0.05), whereas PCr/ATP did not correlate to LV mass index.

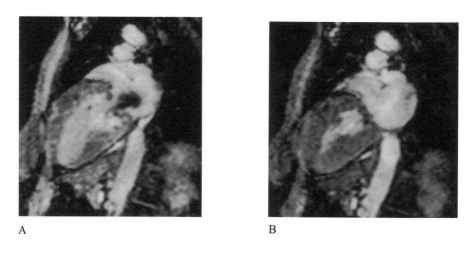

A   B

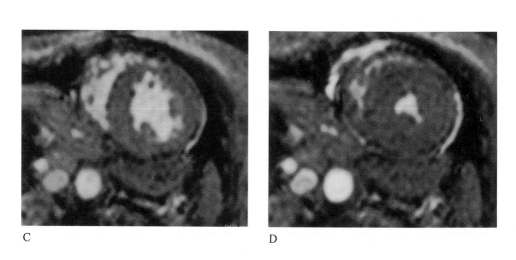

C   D

Figure 8. Two-chamber view at early systole (A) and at end-systole (B) in a patient with aortic valve stenosis (not shown here) and mitral valve insufficiency (shown here). Short-axis images at the papillary muscle level at end-diastole (C) and end-systole (D) show severe LV hypertrophy.

Conclusions

Diastolic LV function and myocardial HEP metabolism are impaired only when LVH is caused by permanent pressure or volume overload, and not by a temporary increase in cardiac workload during part of the day as in elite athletes. Therefore, training-induced and pressure/volume-overload-induced LVH seem to represent different phenotypes of LVH, possibly related to genetic reprogramming which only occurs during permanent cardiac overload.[25] Moreover, there is an association between impaired LV diastolic function and altered myocardial HEP metabolism in patients with hypertension and in patients with aortic valve disease. Finally we did not find a correlation between myocardial HEP metabolism and LV mass in any of the groups studied. The latter indicates that LVH should be regarded as an epiphenomenon to cardiac overload, and not as a primary factor causing abnormal HEP metabolism.

References

1. Levy D, Garrison RJ, Savage DD, Kanel WB, Castelli WP. Prognostic implications of echocardiographically determined left ventricular mass in the Framingham Heart Study. N Engl J Med 1990;322:1561-6.
2. Sadoshima J, Xu Y, Slayter HS, Izumo S. Autocrine release of angiotensin II mediates stretch-induced hypertrophy of cardiac myocytes in vitro. Cell 1993;75:977-84.
3. van Heugten HAA, de Jonge HW, Bezstarosti K, Sharma HS, Verdouw PD, Lamers JMJ. Intracellular signaling and genetic reprogramming during agonist-induced hypertrophy of cardiomyocytes. Ann N Y Acad Sci 1995;752:343-52.
4. Fouad FM, Tarazi RC, Gallagher JH, Macintyre WJ, Cook SA. Abnormal left ventricular relaxation in hypertensive patients. Clin Sci 1980;59:411s-414s.
5. Smith V, Schulman P, Karimeddini MK, White WB, Meeran MK, Katz AM. Rapid ventricular filling in left ventricular hypertrophy: II. Pathologic hypertrophy. J Am Coll Cardiol 1985;5:869-74.
6. Osbakken M, Douglas PS, Ivanics T, Zhang D, Van Winkle T. Creatine kinase kinetics studied by phosphorus-31 nuclear magnetic resonance in a canine model of chronic hypertension-induced cardiac hypertrophy. J Am Coll Cardiol. 1992;19:223-8.
7. Zhang J, Merkle H, Hendrich K, et al. Bioenergetic abnormalities associated with severe left ventricular hypertrophy. J Clin Invest 1993;92:993-1003.
8. Hartiala JJ, Mostbeck GH, Foster E, Fujita N, Dulce MC, Chazouilleres AF, Higgins CB. Velocity-encoded cine MRI in the evaluation of left ventricular diastolic function: measurement of mitral valve and pulmonary vein flow velocities and flow volume across the mitral valve. Am Heart J 1993;125:1054-66.
9. Pattynama PMT, Lamb HJ, van der Velde EA, van der Wall EE, de Roos A. Left ventricular measurements with cine and spin-echo MR imaging: A study of reproducibility with variance component analysis. Radiology 1993;187:261-8.
10. Weiss RG, Bottomley PA, Hardy CJ, Gerstenblith G. Regional myocardial metabolism of high-energy phosphates during isometric exercise in patients with coronary artery disease. N Engl J Med 1990;323:1593-600.
11. Lamb HJ, Doornbos J, den Hollander JA, et al. Reproducibility of human cardiac ^{31}P-NMR spectroscopy. NMR Biomed 1996;9:217-27.
12. Neubauer S, Horn M, Cramer M, et al. Myocardial phosphocreatine-to-ATP ratio is a predictor of mortality in patients with dilated cardiomyopathy. Circulation 1997;96:2190-6.
13. Caputo GR, Suzuki J, Kondo C, et al. Determination of left ventricular volume and mass with use of biphasic spin-echo MR imaging: comparison with cine MR. Radiology 1990;177:773-7.
14. Semelka RC, Tomei E, Wagner S, et al. Normal left ventricular dimensions and function: interstudy reproducibility of measurements with cine MR imaging. Radiology 1990;174:763-8.
15. Tscholakoff D, Higgins CB. Gated magnetic resonance imaging for assessment of cardiac function and myocardial infarction. Radiol Clin North Am 1985;23:449-57.
16. Lamb HJ, Doornbos J, van der Velde EA, Kruit MC, Reiber JHC, de Roos A. Echo planar MRI of the heart on a standard system: validation of measurements of left ventricular function and mass. J Comput Assist Tomogr 1996;20:942-9.
17. Yabe T, Mitsunami K, Okada M, Morikawa S, Inubushi T, Kinoshita M. Detection of myocardial ischemia by 31P magnetic resonance spectroscopy during handgrip exercise. Circulation 1994;89:1709-16.
18. de Roos A, Doornbos J, Luyten PR, Oosterwaal LJMP, van der Wall EE, den Hollander JA. Cardiac metabolism in patients with dilated and hypertrophic cardiomyopathy: Assessment with proton-decoupled P-31 MR spectroscopy. J Magn Reson Imag 1992;2:711-9.
19. Conway MA, Allis J, Ouwerkerk R, Niioka T, Rajagopalan B, Radda GK. Detection of low phosphocreatine to ATP ratio in failing hypertrophied human myocardium by ^{31}P magnetic resonance spectroscopy. Lancet 1991;338:973-6.
20. Bottomley P. MR spectroscopy of the human heart: the status and the challenges. Radiology 1994;191:593-612.
21. Joint National Committee on detection, evaluation, and treatment of high blood pressure. The fifth report of the Joint National Committee on detection, evaluation, and treatment of high blood pressure (JNC V). Arch Intern Med 1993;153:154-83.
22. Lamb HJ, Beyerbacht HP, van der Laarse A, et al. Diastolic dysfunction in hypertensive heart disease is associated with altered myocardial metabolism. Circulation 1999;99:2261-7.
23. Pluim BM, Lamb HJ, Kayser HWM, et al. Functional and metabolic evaluation of the athlete's heart by

magnetic resonance imaging and dobutamine stress magnetic resonance spectroscopy. Circulation 1998;97:666-72.

24. Lamb HJ, Beyerbacht HP, Ouwerkerk R, et al. Metabolic response of normal human myocardium to high-dose atropine-dobutamine stress studied by ^{31}P-MRS. Circulation 1997;96:2969-77.

25. Susic D, Nuñez E, Frohlich ED, Prakash O. Angiotensin II increases left ventricular mass without affecting myosin isoform mRNAs. Hypertension 1996;28:265-8.

9. HYPERTROPHY AND ARRHYTHMIAS

A.A.M. WILDE

Summary

Pathological left ventricular hypertrophy is, regardless of its cause, associated with increased cardiovascular morbidity and mortality. The arrhythmogenic potential is most likely based on several factors, including significant electrophysiological alterations, anatomic alterations (fibrosis) and increased propensity for ischemic events. There is no single responsible arrhythmogenic mechanism. Hence, anti-arrhythmic therapy will be hard to manage successfully. The identification of patients at risk is of critical importance to direct specific therapy, which may include implantation of automatic defibrillators, to those individuals who really need it.

Introduction

Left ventricular hypertrophy is a frequently encountered cardiac abnormality. It is usually associated with hypertensive heart disease, but may also result from congenital malformation(s) or valve disease. In these conditions it can be regarded as an adaptive process by which the heart accommodates to volume overload or increased afterload. In addition, genetic defects in sarcomere function result in ventricular hypertrophy. There is little doubt that cardiac hypertrophy imposes an increased risk for cardiac morbidity and mortality due to an enhanced incidence of (supra-)ventricular arrhythmias, sudden cardiac death, heart failure and myocardial ischemia. This chapter reviews the existing knowledge of arrhythmogeneity of pathological hypertrophy be it either in the setting of hypertensive heart disease or caused by aberrancies in genes encoding sarcomeric proteins.

E. E. van der Wall et al.(eds.), Left Ventricular Hypertrophy, 121-129.
© 1999 *Kluwer Academic Publishers. Printed in the Netherlands.*

Clinical data

There is ample clinical evidence that hypertensive left ventricular hypertrophy is associated with an increased incidence of ventricular arrhythmias. The incidence of complex ventricular arrhythmias, generally defined as ventricular couplets and ventricular tachycardia (= 3 complexes at a rate of 120 beats per minute), has been compared between patients with and without electrocardiographic evidence of hypertensive left ventricular hypertrophy.[1,2] In the second and largest study by McLenachan et al.[2], 48-hour ambulatory electrocardiographic monitoring in 100 treated hypertensive patients revealed a 28% incidence of ventricualr tachycardias in 50 patients with left ventricular hypertrophy compared to 8% in the other 50 without left ventricular hypertrophy (p < 0.05; both groups on comparable treatment and matched for blood pressure level). The presence of ventricular tachycardias or ventricular couplets also differed significantly from 50 age and sex matched controls. Ventricular arrhythmias were more common in patients with hypertrophy accompanied by ST-T-wave changes.[2]

In an attempt to study the prognostic significance of these findings, patients included in the Framingham heart study and Framingham offspring study, with echocardiographic evidence of left ventricular hypertrophy and no clinical evidence of ischemic heart disease had one hour ambulatory ECG monitoring.[3] In a 6-years follow-up period all-cause mortality, cardiac mortality and myocardial infarction was monitored. After adjustment for age and sex, the presence of complex arrhythmias was associated with reduced survival (hazard ratio 1.80, 95% CI: 1.13-2.87, p = 0.013).

In patients with genetically determined hypertrophy data pertinent to prognosis have also been obtained. Hypertrophic cardiomyopathy is a genetically heterogeneous disease with involvement of at least 7 genes, presumably all encoding sarcomeric proteins. Without doubt the presence of sustained ventricular tachycardia or ventricular fibrillation identifies a patient at high risk for sudden cardiac death (for overview see Spirito et al.[4]) The relevance of non-sustained ventricular tachycardias, in particular when they occur infrequently, has heavily been debated over the years. Whereas in the early eighties the presence of single non-sustained ventricular tachycardias warranted amiodarone or other antiarrhythmic drug treatment[5], later studies provided strong evidence that not all of these patients are at high risk.[6] Based on many years of experience of experts in the field, prophylatic antiarrhythmic treatment is currently advised for patients with more than five non-sustained episodes or one episode of more than ten complexes on a single Holter recording.[4] A malignant family history adds to a bad prognosis. Its molecular genetic basis is being unraveled nowadays by the identification of particular 'malignant' mutations in specific genes.[7] Causal involvement of the troponin-T gene seems, regardless of the mutation, always associated with a high incidence of sudden cardiac death.[8] The pathophysiological basis of these differences is not yet known, but it seems likely that the degree of myocardial disarray is of major importance. It should be realized that part of the genotype-phenotype relationship is obtained in untreated families. These data may therefore not be pertinent to currently early diagnosed and optimally treated patients.

In addition to the family history and the ambulatory ECG results, exercise-induced blood pressure alterations seem an important risk factor.[9] A normal blood pressure response, defined as an increase in the systolic pressure of at least 20 mmHg from rest to peak exercise, identifies low risk patients.[9] Finally, invasive electrophysiological techniques in which local right ventricular electrograms are obtained in response to premature stimuli seem to identify patients at risk for sudden cardiac death.[10] Highly fractionated electrograms (i.e. show multiple deflections, a putative reflection of hampered intraventricular conduction) which occur upon relatively late coupled extrasystoles are associated with a bad prognosis.[10] In particular these "fractionation-studies" may prove to be of great benefit in future risk stratification studies.

The pathophysiology of ventricular arrhythmias in hypertensive left ventricular hypertrophy is most likely multifactorial. Electrical instability, based on hypertrophy-induced alterations in action potential morphology, sets the stage for arrhythmias (see next paragraph). In addition, accompanying fibrosis seems to aggravate the electrophysiological abnormalities and may, theoretically, facilitate the induction of (reentrant) arrhythmias.[11] In patients with (genetically) hypertrophic cardiomyopathy the previously discussed clinical electrophysiological studies seem to suggest that conduction disturbances, secondary to myocardial disarray, underlie the arrhythmogenic potential of the disease.

Experimental data

It is important to realize that many experimental models actually represent a mixture of hypertrophy and failure, despite the fact that the experimental environment offers the unique opportunity to distinguish electrophysiological consequences of both processes. On the other hand, in the majority of patients these conditions are combined. Hence, the information obtained may indeed be pertinent to the clinical setting.

Before examining the electrophysiological consequences of cardiac hypertrophy, the basic electrophysiological mechanisms of cardiac arrhythmias will be briefly reviewed. As a general classification, arrhythmias may ensue from abnormalities in impulse initiation or impulse conduction. A subdivision of the first category is formed by automaticity and triggered activity. Automaticity may arise from cardiac cells at a normal resting membrane potential (enhanced normal automaticity) or from cells at a reduced membrane potential (abnormal automaticity). Triggered activity refers to impulse initiation based on afterdepolarizations. Afterdepolarizations are deviations from the normal course of the membrane potential which may occur either during the plateauphase of the action potential (i.e. early afterdepolarizations) or occur during diastole, after completion of the action potential. In either case its occurrence depends on the previous action potential, i.e. is triggered by that particular action potential. The presence of abnormal impulse initiation is not required for reentrant arrhythmias which rely on disturbances in impulse conduction. Under appropriate conditions an electrical impulse may continue to propagate and reexcite tissue that it has previously excited. 'Appropriate conditions' are formed by conduction block and sufficient conduction delay. It will become evident that the electrophysiological abnormalities of hypertrophied tissue favours any arrhythmogenic mechanism.

The characteristic electrophysiological abnormality of hypertrophied tissue is prolongation of the ventricular action potential. Renal hypertension in rats is a frequently used model to study the impact of induced hypertrophy on electrophysiological parameters. Indeed, action potential prolongation has been consistently observed in this model[12-15], as well as in other experimental animal models of cardiac hypertrophy.[11,16-18] However, in human hypertrophied muscle no relation was found between the degree of hypertrophy and the length of the action potential.[19] Whenever it is measured an associated increase in refractory period is found.[18] Other action potential parameters, i.e. resting membrane potential, action potential upstroke and its maximum rate of rise do not change.[11-13,15] Conduction velocity is reduced in a linear fashion with increased degree of hypertrophy, as deduced from cell diameter.[19] The action potential prolongation is definitely more pronounced at a slow heart rate,[14,17] potentially reducing its pathophysiological significance.[20] On the other hand, irregularities in heart rate with consequent long RR intervals are frequently encountered in hypertrophied states. The prolongation may not be uniform and less pronounced in epicardial layers, particularly in the latter half of the action potential.[14] In the epicardial layer itself action potential duration dispersion is also more pronounced in hypertrophied hearts compared to control hearts (Figure 1).[21]

A   B

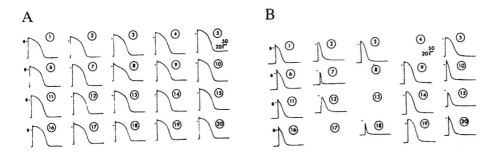

Figure 1. Data taken with courtesy from Cameron et al. (1983) with permission from the author and the publisher. Panel A shows 20 action potential recordings from a 4 mm² surface grid on the anterior papillary muscle in an isolated heart from a control cat (superfused preparation). Action potential duration is fairly homogeneous in all recordings (mean approximately 145 ms). Action potential amplitude is approximately 100 mV.
Panel A shows 20 action potential recordings from a similar grid on a fibrotic region on the anterior anterior papillary muscle of a heart subjected to left ventricular pressure overload by aortic banding several months before this measurement. Note the marked inhomogeneity in action potential morphology and particularly the marked dispersion in action potential duration. At several sites (4,8,13,17) no successful impalement was obtained. Action potential amplitudes are roughly similar and duration is increased to a mean value of 165 ms.

In fibrotic regions of feline hearts subjected to left ventricular pressure overload (aortic banding) marked inhomogeneity in action potential morphology is observed with significant shortening and reduced action potential upstrokes at particular sites.[11] These findings enhance the likelihood that alteration in the action potential shape is causally involved in arrhythmogenesis.Whenever heart failure becomes part of the spectrum, the lengthening of the action potential becomes more pronounced.[17]

The action potential plateau phase is the result of a fine balance between inward (Na^+, Ca^{2+}) and outward (K^+) currents. An increase in net depolarizing (inward) current or a decrease in net repolarizing (outward) current or both will lengthen the action potential. In the past years hypertrophy/heart failure induced alterations in membrane currents have been studied in many different experimental models. There is certainly some consistency in the experimental results (see below), but the intrepretation of the data is hampered by the wide diversity in species and experimental models.A schematic compilation of the data is given in Figure 2. Whereas in heart failure models a decrease in the transient outward current I_{TO} is a consistent finding, it is less clear in hypertrophied states secondary to compensated pressure overload in which even an increase has been reported.[22] Other K^+ currents with more direct impact on the action potential duration, like the fast component of the delayed rectifier,[23,24] may be reduced as well but there is only a limited amount of data. L-type calcium channels appear to be upregulated in experimentals models of hypertrophy and current characteristics are altered in such a way that increased Ca^{2+} current and action potential prolongation ensue. With more severe hypertrophy and heart failure less L-type Ca^{2+} current is commonly observed. An interesting observation is the increase in density of the hyperpolarizing-activated inward Na^+ current I_f.[25]

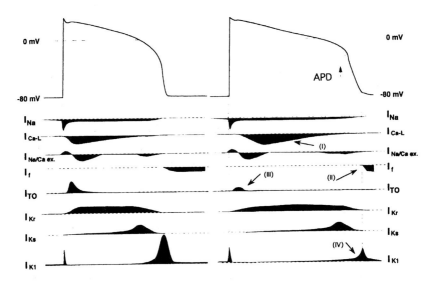

Figure 2. Schematic representation of the ventricular action potential in control conditions (left panel) and in hypertrophy (right panel). Current traces of the main currents are depicted under the action potential traces. The inward currents are presented by a downward deflection and the outward currents by an upward deflection. The amplitude of the trace reflects the relative amplitude of the current during the course of the action potential. I_{Na} is the fast sodium current, I_{CA-L} is the L-type calcium current, $I_{Na/Ca\ ex.}$ is the sodium/calcium exchanger which may generate inward and outward current depending on the voltage level, I_f is the pacemaker current, I_{TO} is the transient outward current, I_{Kr} is the rapid activating component of the delayed rectifier, I_{Ks} is the slow activating component of the delayed rectifier, I_{K1} is the inward rectifier. Hypertrophy-induced changes in ionic currents are shown in the right panel and emphasized by arrows. (I): In most studies an increase in L-type calcium current has been reported. (II): An increase in pacemaker current has been reported. (III): A decrease in the transient outward is not consistently reported and dissociation from failing conditions is not that clear. (IV): A decrease in the inward rectifier may be present.

Theoretically, an increase in action potential duration predisposes to triggered activity based on early afterdepolarizations. Indeed, renal hypertensive dogs are more susceptible to early afterdepolarizations and related ventricular arrhythmias after exposure to 'depolarizing drugs' (blocking K^+ outward current or increasing Ca^{2+} inward current) than control hearts.[18] Similar results were obtained in hypertrophied papillary muscles from renal hypertensive rats.[13] However, in the latter model delayed afterdepolarizations could also be induced under experimental circumstances aimed to increase the intracellular calcium concentration.

In the rat model, attempts to induce early or delayed afterdepolariations in normal myocardium were never successful.[13] In a feline model of cardiac hypertrophy, complex ventricular ectopy was induced upon vagal stimulation in 25% of animals compared to no arrhythmias in control or sham-operated cats.[11]

The appearance of arrhythmias upon slowing of heart rate suggests early afterdepolarizations as the responsible mechanism. However, in this particular model with marked heterogeneity in action potential duration in fibrotic regions, slowing of heart rate may also increase differences in action potential duration, thereby facilitating reentrant arrhythmias. Conduction slowing, as demonstrated in hypertrophied human specimens, similarly increases the likelihood for reentry.[19] Potentially, the increase in I_f enhances abnormal automaticity.[25]

In addition to direct arrhythmogenic consequences of the described (inhomogeneous) action potential alterations, hypertrophic hearts also seem more susceptible to ischemia-related early ventricular arrhythmias.[16] The degree of hypertrophy appeared positively related to the arrhythmogenic susceptibility, but myocardial mass could be excluded as an important determinant.[16] More chronic experiments in dogs also revealed increased 24 and 48 hour mortality after coronary artery occlusion in conscious dogs with hypertensive left ventricular hypertrophy.[26]

Conclusions

Genarally, pathological left ventricular hypertrophy is associated with increased cardiovascular morbidity and mortality. The arrhythmogenic potential is most likely based on several factors, including significant electrophysiological alterations, anatomic

References

1. Messerli FH, Ventura HO, Elizardi DJ, Dunn FG, Frohlich ED. Hypertension and sudden death: increased ventricular ectopic activity in left ventricular hypertrophy. Am J Med 1984;77:18-22.
2. McLenachan JM, Henderson E, Morris KI, Dargie HJ. Ventricular arrhythmias in patients with hypertensive left ventricular hypertrophy. N Engl J Med 1987;317:787-92.
3. Bikkina M, Larson MG, Levy D. Asymptomatic ventricular arrhythmias and mortality risk in subjects with left ventricular hypertrophy. J Am Coll Cardiol 1993;22:1111-6.
4. Spirito P, Seidman CE, McKenna WJ, Maron BJ. The management of hypertrophic cardiomyopathy. N Engl J Med 1997;336:775-82.
5. Maron BJ, Savage DD, Wolfson JK, Epstein SE. Prognostic significance of 24 hour ambulatory electrocardiographic monitoring in patients with hypertrophic cardiomyopathy: a prospective study. Am J Cardiol 1981;48:252- 7.
6. Spirito P, Rapezzi C, Autore C, et al. Prognosis of asymptomatic patients with hypertrophic cardiomyopathy and nonsustained ventricular tachycardia. Circulation 1994;90:2743-7.
7. Schwartz K, Carrier L, Guicheney P, Komajda M. Molecular basis of familial cardiomyopathies. Circulation 1995;91:532-40.
8. Watkins H, McKenna WJ, Thierfelder L, et al. Mutations in the gene for cardiac troponin T and tropomyosin in hyperthrophic cardiomyopathy. N Engl J Med 1995;332:1058-64
9. Sadoul N, Prasad K, Elliott PM, Bannerjee S, Frenneaux MP, McKenna WJ. Prospective prognostic assessment of blood pressure response during exercise in patients with hypertrophic cardiomyopathy. Circulation 1997;96:2987-91.
10. Saumarez RC, Slade AKB, Grace AA, Sadoul N, Camm AJ, McKenna WJ. The significance of paced electrogram fractionation in hypertrophic cardiomyopathy. A prospective study. Circulation 1995;91:2762-8.
11. Cameron JS, Myerburg RJ, Wong SS, et al. Electrophysiologic consequences of chronic experimentally induced left ventricular pressure overload. J Am Coll Cardiol 1983;2:481-7.
12. Gülch RW, Baumann R, Jacob R. Analysis of myocardial action potential in left ventricular hypertrophy of Goldblatt rats. Basic Res Cardiol 1979;74: 769-82.
13. Aronson RS. Afterpotentials and triggered activity in hypertrophied myocardium from rats with renal hypertension. Circ Res 1981;48:720-7.
14. Keung ECH, Aronson RS. Non-uniform electrophysiological properties and electrotonic interaction in hypertrophied rat myocardium.Circ Res 1981;49:150-8.
15. Aronson RS, Nordin C. Electrophysiologic properties of hypertrophied myocytes isolated from rats with renal hypertension. Eur Heart J 1984;5 Suppl F: 339-45.
16. Kohya T, Kimuara S, Myerburg RJ, Bassett AL. Susceptibility of hypertrophied rat hearts to ventricular fibrillation during acute ischemia. J Mol Cell Cardiol 1988;20:159-68.
17. Nordin C, Siri F, Aronson RS. Electrophysiologic characteristics of single myocytes isolated from hypertrophied guinea-pig hearts. J Mol Cell Cardiol 1989; 21:729-39.
18. Ben-David J, Zipes DP, Ayers GM, Pride HP. Canine left ventricular hypertrophy predisposes to ventricular tachycardia induction by phase 2 early afterdepolarizations after administration of BAY K 8644. J Am Coll Cardiol 1992; 20: 1576-84.
19. McIntyre H, Fry CH. Abnormal action potential conduction in isolated human hypertrophied left ventricular myocardium. J Cardiovasc Electrophysiol 1997;8:887-94.
20. Vermeulen JT. Mechanisms of arrhythmias in heart failure. J Cardiovasc Electrophysiol 1998;9:208-21.
21. Gillis AM, Mathison HJ, Kulisz E, Lester WM. Dispersion of ventricular repolarization in left ventricular hypertrophy: Influence of afterload and dofetilide. J Cardiovasc Electrophysiol 1998;9:988-97.
22. Li Q, Keung EC. Effects of myocardial hypertrophy on transient outward current. Am J Physiol 1994; 266:H1738-45.
23. Kleiman RB, Houser SR. Outward currents in normal and hypertrophied feline ventricular myocytes. Am J Physiol 1989; 256:H1450-61
24. Furukawa T, Myerburg RJ, Furukawa N, Kimura S, Bassett AL. Metabolic inhibition of I_{Ca-L} and I_K differs in feline left ventricular hypertrophy. Am J Physiol 1994; 266:H1121-31.
25. Cerbai E, Barbieri M, Mugelli A. Occurrence and properties of the hyperpolarization-activated current I_f in ventricular myocytes from normotensive and hypertensive rats during aging. Circulation 1996;94:1674-81.
26. Koyanagi S, Eastham C, Marcus ML. Effects of chronic hypertension and left ventricular hypertrophy on the incidence of sudden cardiac death after coronary artery occlusion in conscious dogs.Circulation 82;65:1192-7.

of supraventricular tachycardia was expected to occur during therapy with calcium antagonists, the 74% reduction of ventricular ectopy and the complete suppression of ventricular couplets, multiform contractions and more complex ventricular arrhythmias were unexpected. These results were considered to be specific for LVH and could already be observed during regression of LVH. The latter is accompanied by an improvement of subendocardial ischemia and improvement of electrical irritability of the hypertrophic myocardium. Lowering of arterial blood pressure *per se* could not be the explanation of the anti-arrhythmic efficacy of calcium-antagonists, as diuretic therapy reduced blood pressure to the same extent. In a 4-year antihypertensive therapy study that included 304 patients, 60 endpoints in 54 patients had been recorded: 17 strokes, 13 myocardial infarctions, 30 patients with coronary insufficiency, and 8 deaths[11]. In the group without complications LV mass had decreased by 30±3 g, whereas in the group with complications LV mass had not changed during 4 years of therapy (+0.3±8.3 g). If all patients were divided into 3 groups, group 1 with regression of LV mass, group 2 showing no change in LV mass, and group 3 with LVH progression, a statistically greater incidence of complications occurred in group 3, as compared to the other two groups. These complications were coronary insufficiency (p<0.0007), death (p<0.005), all complications (p<0.0001), and a tendency toward myocardial infarction (p=0.061). This result was confirmed by Koren et al.[12], who reported that hypertensive patients who has decreased or unchanged LV mass index upon 5.3 years of antihypertensive therapy had less cardiovascular events than those who had LVH progression (6% *vs.* 16%, respectively).

Muiesan et al.[13] studied 151 hypertensive patients during long-term antihypertensive therapy. Echocardiographic examination was performed twice with a mean interval of 10 years. Patients without regression of LVH had higher incidence of non-fatal cardiovascular events compared to patients with regression of LVH. The latter group had a significantly reduced risk which almost normalized by complete regression of LVH. To summarize, risk reduction by reversal of LVH appears independent of blood pressure lowering.

Reversal of LVH: association with reversal of myocardial fibrosis?

Brilla et al.[14] treated spontaneously hypertensive rats with the ACE-inhibitor lisinopril for 8 months. Normalization of arterial blood pressure and complete reversal of LVH were associated with reversal of myocardial fibrosis. The latter was related to improvement of diastolic stiffness and systolic stress-strain relations of the left ventricle. Reduction of myocardial fibrosis was considered to be due to enhanced collagen degradation by activation of myocardial matrix metalloproteinase-1. Consequently, reversal of LVH appears to be associated with reversal of myocardial fibrosis.

Risk reduction: lowering blood pressure or reducing LV mass?

Evidence from in vivo, in vitro, and genetic studies suggested that the development as well as the reversal of LVH do not depend solely on hemodynamic load but also on other factors.[15] Several humoral agents that may affect mitogenesis of cardiac myocytes and nonmyocytic elements have been identified, including angiotensin-II, norepinephrine, endothelins, transforming growth factor β, insuline-like growth factor, prostaglandins and nitric oxide. Interference with these mechanisms will restore -at least partly- the normal muscular phenotype and will reduce the risks associated with LVH. Interventions that are aimed to counteract these trophic mechanisms, such as ACE-inhibitors or angiotensin-II antagonists, may contribute to regression of LVH. Bruckschlegel et al.,[16] who used a rat model with pressure overload LVH through banding the ascending aorta, showed that ACE-inhibitors, but not hydralazine, induced LVH reversal in the absence of relief of ventricular afterload, indicating that also other factors were involved. Therefore, regression of vascular hypertrophy and increase of arterial compliance will reduce pulsatile load to the heart and in turn contribute to regression of LVH. Consequently, reduction of LV mass *per se*, independent of lowering blood pressure, may be effective in reducing risk.

Reversal of LVH: new antihypertensive drugs?

Until now, ACE-inhibitors have been shown most effective in reducing LVH. Recently, clinical studies have shown that losartan, a selective angiotensin-II receptor type 1 antagonist, may have profound effects on cardiac hypertrophy as well.[17-19] In a review article from 1995,[18] Dahlöf addressed the advantages of angiotensin-II antagonists in counteracting LVH. It was suggested that losartan exerts its beneficial effects on increased LV mass by inhibition of protein synthesis in cardiac myocytes and increasing endothelin synthesis in the vascular wall. Cuspidi et al.[19] showed in 17 patients with hypertension that losartan significantly reduced LV mass after 6 months of treatment. In this study, the effect on blood pressure lowering by losartan was similar to verapamil, but only losartan induced reduction of LV mass. Recently, Tedesco et al.[20] showed in 33 hypertensive patients that losartan significantly reduced LV wall mass compared to hydrochlorothiazide after 22 months of treatment; LV wall mass normalized in even 30% of patients. The hypothesis that angiotensin-II antagonists offer long-term advantages in hypertensive LVH is currently being tested in the LIFE study (Losartan Intervention For Endpoint reduction in hypertension). The LIFE study comprises 9194 patients who have been randomized to losartan or atenolol and followed for at least 4 years (through April 2001) to accumulate the necessary number of cardiovascular fatal and non-fatal events (minimum of 1040 patients).[21]

Conclusions

In hypertensive patients with LVH, antihypertensive therapy should be targeted to reduce LV mass with the purpose to restore normal muscular phenotype, normalize coronary flow reserve, improve vascular compliance and diminish myocardial fibrosis. As risk reduction by LVH reversal appears independent of blood pressure lowering, antihypertensive therapy should become focused on "antihypertrophic" therapy. At present, ACE-inhibitors appear to be more potent than β-blockers, calcium-antagonists and diuretics in reducing LV mass. There are, in addition, novel drugs that could play a major role in reversal of LVH such as angiotensin-II receptor antagonists, renin inhibitors, L-arginine, sex hormones, and potassium-channel openers.[22]

Future long-term trials are needed (and already underway) [21,23] to elucidate important issues such as the most effective drugs in regression of LVH, whether complete normalization of LV mass should be the goal of antihypertensive therapy, and whether reversal of LVH would favorably change the diagnosis of the hypertensive patient.

References

1. Levy D, Garrison RJ, Savage DD, Kannel WB, Castelli WP. Prognostic implications of echocardiographicly determined left ventricular mass in the Framingham heart study. N Engl J Med 1990;322:1561-6.
2. Levy D, Garrison RJ, Savage DD et al. Left ventricular mass and incidence of coronary heart disease in an elderly cohort: the Framingham Heart Study. Ann Intern Med 1989;110:101-7.
3. Haider AW, Larson MG, Benjamin EJ, Levy D. Increased left ventricular mass and hypertrophy are associated with increased risk for sudden death. J Am Coll Cardiol 1998;32:1454-9.
4. Levy D, Anderson KM, Plehn J, Savage DD, Christiansen JC, Castelli WP. Echocardiographically determined left ventricular structural and functional correlates of complex or frequent ventricular arrhythmias on one-hour ambulatory echocardiographic monitoring. Am J Cardiol 1987;59:836-40.
5. Cruickshank J, Lewis J, Moore V, Dodd C. Reversibility of left ventricular hypertrophy of different types of antihypertensive therapy. J Hum Hypertens 1992;6:85-90.
6. Dahlöf B, Pennert K, Hansson L. Reversal of left ventricular hypertrophy in hypertensive patients. A meta-analysis of 109 treatment studies. Am J Hypertens 1992;5:95-110.
7. Schmieder RE, Martus P, Klingbeil A. Reversal of left ventricular hypertrophy in essential hypertension: a meta-analysis of randomized double-blind studies. JAMA 1996;275:1507-13.
8. Collins R, Peto R, MacMahon S et al. Blood pressure, stroke, and coronary heart disease. Part 2. Short-term reductions in blood pressure: overview of randomized drug trials in their epidemiological context. Lancet 1990;335:827-38.
9. Messerli FH, Nunez BD, Nunez MM, Garavaglia GE, Schmieder RE, Ventura HO. Hypertension and sudden death. Disparate effects of calcium entry blocker and diuretic therapy on cardiac dysrhythmias. Arch Intern Med 1989;149:1263-7.
10. Franz IW, Tönnesmann U, Müller JFM. Time course of complete normalization of left ventricular hypertrophy during long-term antihypertensive therapy with angiotensin converting enzyme inhibitors. Am J Hypertens 1998;11:631-9.
11. Yurenev AP, Dyakonova, Novikov ID et al. Management of essential hypertension in patients with different degrees of left ventricular hypertrophy. Am J Hypertens 1992;5:182S-189S.
12. Koren MJ, Ulin RJ, Laragh JH, Devereux RB. Reduction in left ventricular mass during treatment of essential hypertension is associated with improved prognosis. Am J Hypertens 1991;4:1A (Abstract).
13. Muiesan ML, Salvetti M, Rizzoni D et al. Association of change in left ventricular mass with prognosis during long-term antihypertensive treatment. J Hypertens 1995;13:1091-5.
14. Brilla CG, Matsubara L, Weber KT. Advanced hypertensive heart disease in spontaneously hypertensive rats. Lisinopril-mediated regression of myocardial fibrosis. Hypertension 1996;28:269-75.
15. Susic D, Nunez E, Frohlich ED. Reversal of hypertrophy: an active process. Curr Opin Cardiol 1995;10:466-72.
16. Bruckschlegel G, Holmer SR, Jandeleit K et al. Blockade of the renin-angiotensin system in cardiac pressure-overload hypertrophy in rats. Hypertension 1995;25:250-9.
17. Maisch B, Brilla C, Kruse T. Directions in antihypertensive treatment—our future from the past. Eur Heart J 1995;16 (Suppl C):74-85.
18. Dahlöf B. Effect of angiotension II blockade on cardiac hypertrophy and remodelling: a Review. J Hum Hypertens 1995;9 (Suppl 5):S37-44.
19. Cuspidi C, Lonati L, Sampieri L et al. Effects of losartan on blood pressure and left ventricular mass in essential hypertension. High Blood Press 1998;7:75-9.
20. Tedesco MA, Ratti G, Aquino D et al. Effects of losartan on hypertension and left ventricular mass: a long-term study. J Human Hypertens 1999;12:505-10.
21. Dahlöf B, Devereux RB, Julius S et al. Characteristics of 9194 patients with left ventricular hypertrophy: the LIFE study. Losartan Intervention For Endpoint reduction in Hypertension. Hypertension 1998;32:989-97.
22. Morgan TO, Delbridge IM. Angiotensin blocking drugs and the heart beyond 2000. J Am Soc Nephrol 1999;10 (Suppl 11):S243-7.
23. Devereux RB, Dahlöf B, Levy D, Pfeffer MA. Comparison of enalapril versus nifedipine to decrease left ventricular hypertrophy in systemic hypertension (the PRESERVE trial). Am J Cardiol 1996;78:61-5.

11. POSTOPERATIVE REGRESSION OF LEFT VENTRICULAR HYPERTROPHY

L.H.B. Baur, J. Braun, A.P. Kappetein, C.H. Peels, X.Y. Jin, Y. Houdas, E.A. van der Velde, M. Hazekamp, E.E. van der Wall, A.V.G. Bruschke, H.A. Huysmans

Summary

Long lasting valvular heart disease can result in damage to the cardiac muscle. However, if valve surgery is performed before the ventricular myocardium has been irreversibly damaged, myocardial structure and function will return to normal. If the valvular defect is repaired too late, left ventricular dysfunction will persist. Specific changes of left ventricular function and regression of left ventricular hypertrophy are dependent on the affected valve, the type of valve disease and the duration of valvular disease. In the current chapter, postoperative regression of left ventricular hypertrophy is described for aortic valve stenosis, aortic insuffiency and mitral valve regurgitation.

Introduction

Long lasting valvular disease has considerable impact on left ventricular chamber geometry and myocardial function. Changes in left ventricular function, volume and mass are dependent on the responsible valve, and the disease state (stenosis or insufficiency). If the valve defect is corrected before the left ventricular myocardium has been irreversibly damaged, myocardial structure and function will ultimately return to normal. However, if valvular disease is corrected too late, left ventricular dysfunction will persist. Changes of ventricular geometry and mass differ for the various disease entities and will therefore be discussed separately.

E. E. van der Wall et al.(eds.), Left Ventricular Hypertrophy, 139-150.
© 1999 *Kluwer Academic Publishers. Printed in the Netherlands.*

Aortic valve stenosis

Aortic valve stenosis is associated with chronic pressure overload. In patients with aortic valve stenosis in the compensated stage, this process is accompanied by an adaptive increase in left ventricular mass with a preserved left ventricular enddiastolic volume and stroke volume.[1,2] Ventricular hypertrophy in aortic valve stenosis involves both the muscular and nonmuscular compartments of the left ventricle[3] and is assumed to result from parallel addition of new myofibrils[4] and an increase of interstitial tissue. The gain of left ventricular muscle and interstitial tissue will initially result in diastolic dysfunction.[3] Longstanding severe pressure or volume overload, however, will ultimately lead to myocardial depression with reduced stroke volume but still no irreversible myocardial damage.[20] This process, also known as *"afterload mismatch"*[5] can readily be reversed by lowering afterload. If aortic valve disease is not corrected in this stage, irreversible myocardial damage may occur with persistent left ventricular dysfunction even if the aortic valve has been replaced. Characteristic differences in evolution of left ventricular function and left ventricular hypertrophy in patients with aortic valve stenosis have been reported between women and men. Women with aortic valve stenosis have a characteristic pattern of concentric left ventricular hypertrophy with a smaller, thicker-walled chamber compared with an eccentric pattern of hypertrophy and chamber dilation observed in men.[6] With similar degrees of left ventricular outflow obstruction, cardiac performance is frequently more reduced in men than in women.[6]

Preoperative left ventricular function and the pattern of left ventricular hypertrophy have been shown to be the most important determinants of survival among patients undergoing aortic valve replacement.[7,8] Aortic valve surgery results in immediate reduction in preload and afterload.[9] In most patients, improvement of left ventricular function and regression of left ventricular hypertrophy will occur.[10] This process starts immediately after operation and may continue for decades after surgical intervention.[11] It has been reported that females show a better recovery of left ventricular hypertrophy than males.[12] The lower transvalvular gradients associated with homografts and stentless valves could result in a more complete regression of left ventricular hypertrophy than has been observed with mechanical prostheses or stented bioprostheses.[13] Although some authors found a greater reduction of left ventricular mass in patients with a stentless valve compared to stented bioprostheses,[14] others were not able to confirm this finding.[15,16] Only large clinical trials comparing stented bioprosthetic valves, stentless bioprosthetic valves, and mechanical valves in relation to survival, clinical status and regression of left ventricular hypertrophy will solve this issue. Although regression of left ventricular hypertrophy is prominent in most patients after valve replacement, several factors can disturb this process. Left ventricular mass is known to increase with age,[17,18] with an even larger increase in females compared to males.[19] The presence of hypertension may inhibit complete regression of left ventricular hypertrophy.

Aortic insufficiency

Aortic valve insufficiency is associated with left ventricular volume overload. If aortic valve disease is not corrected, patients with aortic regurgitation follow a predictable course, which is characterized by progressive left ventricular dilation and left ventricular dysfunction.[20] In patients with compensated aortic insufficiency left ventricular enddiastolic volume, stroke volume and left ventricular mass will be increased, whereas left ventricular ejection fraction remains normal.[2,20] In patients with decompensated aortic insufficiency left ventricular end-diastolic volume, stroke volume and mass will be increased, whereas left ventricular ejection fraction remains normal. The increase in left ventricular volume and mass is due to both parallel and series addition of new myofibrils in the ventricular myocardium.[4] After aortic valve replacement left ventricular dimension and left ventricular mass decreases in most patients within six months.[21] However, some patients will have persistent symptoms of congestive heart failure even if the after the aortic valve has been replaced.[22] These patients can be identified by a preoperative fractional shortening measured with echocardiography < 25% , an enddiastolic diameter > 38 mm/m^2 or an endsystolic dimension > 26 mm/m.[2,21,23] These patients may fail to show any improvement in left ventricular function or decrease of left ventricular mass after aortic valve surgery.

Own experience in patients with aortic valve disease

Our experience consists of the combined data-set of patients, who received a Freestyle stentless aortic bioprosthesis in Leiden, the Netherlands; Oxford, United Kingdom; Lille, France; and Eindhoven, the Netherlands. Between June 1993 and June 1998, 240 patients, who received a Freestyle stentless bioprosthesis were echocardiographically examined four weeks after aortic valve replacement and 3-6 months, one year, and two years after aortic valve replacement. Follow-up was complete in 167 patients after 3-6 months, in 180 patients after one year, and in 108 patients after two years. Mean age of the patient group was 68 years. Echocardiograms were made according to the guidelines proposed by the American Society of Echocardiography. Examinations included a M-Mode tracing, a two-dimensional echocardiogram in apical four- and five-chamber view, a pulsed Doppler recording of the left ventricular outflow velocities, and a continuous wave Doppler recording of the aortic valve velocities. Additionally, a color-flow Doppler image was performed from the parasternal long axis view and the apical view. Left ventricular mass was calculated using M-Mode measurements of wall thickness and left ventricular enddiastolic diameter according to the formula: Mass = $1.04[(IVSd+LVDd+PWd)^3 - (LVDd)^3] -13.6$. In this formula IVSd = interventricular septum at diastole, PWd = posterior wall at diastole, and LVDd = left ventricular dimension at diastole. Left ventricular volume was calculated according to the formula given by Teichholz: Diastolic volume = $7 \times (LVDd^3))/2.4 + LVDd)$. Shortening fraction was calculated as (LVDd-LVDs)/LVDd x 100%.

In the present study, the mean gradient across the Freestyle xenograft was low: 7.9 ± 5.1 mmHg at discharge, decreasing to 5.5 mmHg after 3-6 months, 5.4 ± 3.7 mmHg after 1 year and 5.0 ± 3.5 mmHg after two years. The cardiac index was stable at 2.9 ± 1.0 l/min/m^2 throughout the study period. Aortic valve insufficiency grade 1 was present in 9.8% of the patients, and grade 2 in 0.9% of the patients. All these patients had a paravalvular leakage.

Left ventricular mass was 170.6 ± 72.3 g/m^2 within four weeks after valve replacement which decreased to 143.6 ± 55.2 g/m^2 after 3-6 months, 135.6 ± 61.2 g/m^2 after one year, and 133.5 ± 50.5 g/m^2 after two years (p<0.001). Left ventricular volume index remained stable and was 62.2 ± 30.2 ml/m^2 four weeks after surgery, 59.7 ± 24.5 ml/m^2 3-6 months after surgery, 62.9 ± 34.5 ml/m^2 one year after surgery, and 62.6 ± 20.9 ml/m^2 two years after surgery.

Left ventricular ejection fraction increased from 54.2 ± 17.7% four weeks after operation to 58.6 ± 15.4% 3-6 months after surgery, 61.2 ± 15.9% one year after operation, and 59.8 ± 14.3% two years after operation (p<0.001).

Influence of etiology on left ventricular remodeling

We found different strata of left ventricular remodeling in patients with pure valve aortic stenosis, pure aortic insufficiency and combined aortic valve disease (Table 1-3).

Pure aortic valve stenosis (a preoperative transvalvular gradient more than 50 mmHg without aortic insufficiency) was present in 67% of the patient population (Table 1). Mean transvalvular gradient across the Freestyle valve was 8.5 ± 5.4 mmHg within four weeks after operation and decreased to 5.4 ± 3.9 mmHg two years after operation ($p < 0.0001$). Left ventricular ejection fraction was 53.4 ± 18.1 % within one month after operation and increased to 61.6 ± 13.0 % ($p<0.0001$). Left ventricular mass index was 170.8 ± 66.8 g/m^2 at discharge and decreased to 122.0 ± 44.5 g/m^2 after two years ($p<0.0001$). This meant a regression of left ventricular mass of 29%. It was obvious, that this patient group left ventricular function improved and left ventricular hypertrophy diminished considerably.

Pure aortic insufficiency (aortic insufficiency more than grade 2, without an increased transvalvular gradient) was present in 18% of patients (Table 2). In these patients, mean postoperative transvalvular gradient across the Freestyle valve was 7.2 ± 4.4 mmHg which decreased to 4.9 ± 3.2 mmHg after two years ($p<0.005$). Left ventricular ejection fraction improved from 47.1 ± 20.5% to 60.9 ± 19.6% after two years ($p<0.0001$). Left ventricular mass index was higher early postoperative at 196.7 ± 74.4 g/m^2 and showed a far less important decrease to 179.3 ± 63.1 g/m^2 after two years ($p<0.01$). Decrease of left ventricular hypertrophy was only 10% in this patient group. In 15% of the patients combined aortic valve disease (aortic valve stenosis and insufficiency) was present (Table 3). In these patients the transvalvular gradient across the Freestyle valve was 6.0 ± 3.7 mmHg after operation which decreased to 4.0 ± 2.7 mmHg after 2 years ($p< 0.001$). Left ventricular ejection fraction was 55.0 ± 14.9% within some weeks after operation and remained the same (56.7 ± 11.7%) after two years. However, left ventricular mass index decreased to the same extent as was observed in patients with aortic valve stenosis, namely from 165.2 ± 67.7 g/m^2 to 128.2 ± 38.9 g/m^2 ($p<0.01$).

Table 1. Mean transvalvular gradients across the stentless aortic bioprosthesis, cardiac index, left ventricular volumes, left ventricular mass and left ventricular ejection fraction during two years follow-up after aortic valve replacement in patients with preoperative aortic valve stenosis.

	< 4 weeks post surgery	3-6 months post surgery	1 year post surgery	2 years post surgery	p value
No. of pts	161	108	123	72	
Mean valvular gradient (mmHg)	8.5 ± 5.4	5.4 ± 3.4	5.3 ± 3.8	5.4 ± 3.9	<0.0001
Cardiac index (l/min/m²)	2.8 ± 0.9	2.8 ± 1.0	2.9 ± 0.9	2.9 ± 1.1	NS
LVEDV index (ml/m²)	60.2 ± 26.6	60.4 ± 25.0	66.4 ± 39.3	57.6 ± 17.8	NS
LV mass index (g/m²)	170.8 ± 66.8	144.8 ± 55.3	136.9 ± 67.7	122.0 ± 44.5	<0.0001
LVEF (%)	53.4 ± 18.1	58.7 ± 14.9	61.1 ± 16.0	61.6 ± 13.1	<0.0001

Table 2. Mean transvalvular gradients across the stentless aortic bioprosthesis, cardiac index, left ventricular volumes, left ventricular mass and left ventricular ejection fraction during two years follow-up after aortic valve replacement in patients with preoperative aortic valve insufficiency.

	< 4 weeks post surgery	3-6 months post surgery	1 year post surgery	2 years post surgery	p value
No. of pts	44	21	21	18	
Mean valvular gradient (mmHg)	7.2 ± 4.4	3.4 ± 2.6	4.5 ± 3.4	5.1 ± 3.2	<0.0001
Cardiac index (l/min/m²)	3.2 ± 1.3	3.1 ± 1.1	3.1 ± 0.9	3.2 ± 0.8	NS
LVEDV index (ml/m²)	76.6 ± 35.9	70.5 ± 24.7	65.1 ± 26.5	71.8 ± 26.6	NS
LV mass index (ml/m²)	196.7 ± 74.4	150.7 ± 60.3	145.7 ± 56.4	179.3 ± 63.1	<0.01
LVEF (%)	47.1 ± 20.4	52.2 ± 14.0	57.4 ± 15.8	62.1 ± 19.7	< 0.05

Table 3. Mean transvalvular gradients across the stentless aortic bioprosthesis, cardiac index, left ventricular volumes, left ventricular mass and left ventricular ejection fraction during two years follow-up after aortic valve replacement in patients with preoperative aortic valve disease (combined).

	< 4 weeks post surgery	3-6 months post surgery	1 year post surgery	2 years post surgery	p value
No. of pts	44	38	36	28	
Mean valvular gradient (mmHg)	6.0 ± 3.7	4.2 ± 2.4	4.5 ± 2.7	4.0 ± 2.7	< 0.005
Cardiac index (l/min/m²)	2.9 ± 1.0	2.6 ± 0.7	2.7 ± 0.7	2.7 ± 0.9	NS
LVEDV index (ml/m²)	68.3 ± 33.1	68.5 ± 24.7	61.6 ± 23.4	64.9 ± 17.4	NS
LV mass Index (ml/m²)	165.3 ± 67.7	139.2 ± 47.2	125.4 ± 54.5	128.2 ± 38.9	< 0.001
LVEF (%)	55.0 ± 14.9	56.9 ± 14.7	60.5 ± 14.8	56.7 ± 11.7	NS

Table 4. Mean transvalvular gradients across the stentless aortic bioprosthesis, cardiac index, left ventricular volumes, left ventricular mass and left ventricular ejection fraction during two years follow-up in patients with and without coronary artery disease.

	Coronary Artery Disease present < 4 weeks post surgery	Coronary Artery Disease absent < 4 weeks post surgery	Coronary Artery Disease present 2 years post surgery	Coronary Artery Disease absent 2 years post surgery	*p value* Presence versus Absence Coronary Artery Disease
No. of pts	94	161	53	72	
Mean valvular gradient (mmHg)	8.4 ± 5.3	7.4 ± 5.1	4.8 ± 2.7	5.1 ± 3.9	NS
Cardiac index (l/min/m²)	2.9 ± 1.0	2.8 ± 1.0	2.9 ± 0.9	2.9 ± 1.1	NS
LVEDV index (ml/m²)	63.1 ± 28.3	63.8 ± 31.7	65,1 ± 22,8	60.9 ± 19.1	NS
LV mass Index (ml/m²)	184.3 ± 75.6	167.3 ± 68.5	144.8 ± 53.2	124.2 ± 46.1	<0.02
LVEF (%)	48.6 ± 19.9	58.7 ± 14.9	54.6 ± 16.8	61.2 ± 13.8	NS

Although no complete information was available about left ventricular function before valve replacement, the following conclusions can be made.

Left ventricular mass decreased both in patients with aortic valve stenosis and in patients with aortic insufficiency. However, the extent of left ventricular remodeling was larger in patients with aortic valve stenosis. Recovery of left ventricular function was observed both in patients with aortic valve stenosis and aortic valve insufficiency, but was absent in patients with combined aortic valve disease.

Influence of concomitant coronary artery disease on left ventricular remodeling

The influence of concomitant coronary artery disease on left ventricular remodeling can be derived from Table 4. Patients with coronary artery disease, which was defined as a more than 50% luminal stenosis in one of the epicardial coronary arteries, showed equal transvalvular gradients, and equal left ventricular ejection fraction and left ventricular volumes during 2 years follow-up. However, early postoperative left ventricular mass index was higher in patients with coronary artery disease and decreased less than in those patients without significant coronary artery disease (p<0.02).

Mitral valve insufficiency

Mitral valve regurgitation exposes the left ventricle to an excessive volume load, leading to a series of compensatory myocardial and circulatory adjustments.[24,25] Initially, volume overload is associated with an increase of left ventricular enddiastolic volume and left ventricular mass, bur with preserved left ventricular contractility.[26] Because of the low impedance of the ejection into the left atrium, afterload is reduced. This reduction in afterload allows endsystolic volume and ejection fraction to remain near-normal.[27] When severe mitral insufficiency persists, the left ventricle dilates considerably. The progressive left ventricular dilation increases systolic wall stress and endsystolic volume with a diminished left ventricular function.[28,29] Dilation of the mitral annulus results in a further increased severity of mitral insufficiency and progressive deterioration of left ventricular function. After some time left ventricular dysfunction becomes irreversible despite surgical correction of the mitral valve.[30] It is therefore not suprising that preoperative left ventricular function has been identified as the most important predictor of postoperative outcome after mitral valve surgery.[31]

In the clinical situation and in clinical studies, left ventricular function is frequently measured by left ventricular ejection fraction. However, left ventricular ejection fraction is afterload dependent[32] and often remains higher than expected, thereby masking the presence of left ventricular dysfunction.[33] Measurement of the maximal elastance at endsystole will reflect better left ventricular performance because this is less dependent on changes in afterload.[34] After mitral valve replacement left ventricular ejection fraction will often drop due to an increase in systolic wall stress.[35]

Two groups of patients, who will perform differently after operation, can be identified.[35,36]

In the first group, preoperative echocardiographically measured left ventricular endsystolic dimension is lower than 26 mm/m^2 and left ventricular shortening fraction is higher than 31%. In these patients, enddiastolic dimension and left ventricular mass decrease after mitral valve repair or mitral valve replacement with a slight decrease in ejection fraction. In the second group with a severely enlarged left ventricle and a left ventricular endsystolic dimension > 26 mm/m^2 or a left ventricular shortening fraction < 31%, left ventricular dimensions and mass do not reduce after repair or substitution of the mitral valve. However, following operation, left ventricular ejection fraction drops dramatically in this group. In addition, these patients will remain symptomatic despite surgery.

Besides the preoperative myocardial status, mechanical integrity of the mitral apparatus appears to be another important factor in preservation of postoperative left ventricular function. Patients whose mitral apparatus is left intact will show minimal reduction in left ventricular ejection fraction, whereas patients in whom the mitral valve is completely excised show a significant reduction in postoperative left ventricular ejection fraction.[37] Consequently, mitral valvuloplasty is superior to valve replacement for preservation of left ventricular function after mitral valve surgery.

Conclusions

Regression of left ventricular hypertrophy due to valvular disease will occur if damage of the left ventricular myocardium is not too advanced. Therefore, early surgery is warranted.

Conservative surgery and *"physiologic valve replacement with homografts or stentless valves"* result in a better recovery of left ventricular function than valve replacement with mechanical valves.

References

1. Kennedy JW, Doces J, Stewart DK. Left ventricular function before and following aortic valve replacement. Circulation 1977;56:944-50.
2. Krayenbuehl HP, Hess OM, Monrad S, Schneider J, Mall G, Turina M. Left ventricular myocardial structure in aortic valve disease before, intermediate, and late after aortic valve replacement. Circulation 1989;79:744-55.
3. Schwarz F, Flameng W, Schaper J, Hehrlein F. Correlation between myocardial structure and diastolic properties of the heart in chronic aortic valve disease: Effects of corrective surgery. Am J Cardiol 1976;42:895-903.
4. Grossman W. Cardiac hypertrophy: useful adaptation or pathologic process? Am J Med 1980;69:576-84.
5. Ross J. Jr. Afterload mismatch and preload reserve: a conceptual framework for the analysis of ventricular function. Prog Cardiovasc Dis 1976;18:255-64.
6. Caroll JD, Caroll EP, Feldman T et al. Sex-associated differences in left ventricular function in aortic stenosis in the elderly. Circulation 1992;86:1099-107.
7. Morris JJ, Schaff HV, Mullany CJ et al. Determinants of survival and recovery of left ventricular function after aortic valve replacement. Ann Thorac Surg 1993;56:22-30.
8. Orsinelli DA, Aurigemma GP, Battista S, Krendel S, Gaasch WH. Left ventricular hypertrophy and mortality after aortic valve replacement for aortic stenosis. J Am Coll Cardiol 1993;22:1679-83.
9. Harpole DH, Jones RH. Serial assessment of ventricular performance after valve replacement for aortic stenosis. J Thorac Cardiovasc Surg 1990;99:645-50.
10. Pantely G, Morton M, Rahimtoola SH. Severe aortic stenosis with impaired left ventricular function and clinical heart failure: results of valve replacement. Circulation 1978;58:255-64.
11. Monrad ES, Hess OM, Murakami T, Nonogi H, Corin WJ, Krayenbuel HP. Abnormal exercise hemodynamics in patients with normal systolic function late after valve replacement. Circulation 1988;77:613-24.
12. Morris JJ, Schaff HV, Mullany CJ, Morris PB, Frye RL, Orszulak TA. Gender differences in left ventricular function response to aortic valve replacement. Circulation 1994;90:{part 2):II-183-II-189.
13. Baur LHB, Braun J, Peels CH et al. Haemodynamics of the Freestyle stentless aortic bioprosthesis. Cardiologie 1998;5:555-61.
14. Jin XY, Zhong ZM, Gibson DG, Yacoub MH, Pepper JR. Effects of valve substitute on changes in left ventricular function and hypertrophy after aortic valve replacement. Ann Thorac Cardiovasc Surg 1996;62:1084-9.
15. Christakis GT, Joyner CD, Morgan CD et al. Left ventricular mass regression early after aortic valve replacement. Ann Thorac Surg 1996;62:1084-9.
16. De Paulis R, Sommariva L, Colagrande L et al. Regression of left ventricular hypertrophy after aortic valve replacement for aortic stenosis with different valve substitutes. J Thorac Cardiovasc Surg 1998;116:590-8.
17. Messerli FH, Clinical determinants and manifestations of left ventricular hypertrophy. In: Messerli FH, editors. The Heart and Hypertension. New York: Yorke Medical Books;1987; p. 219-30.
18. Lindroos M, Kupari M, Heikkila J, Tilvis R. Echocardiographic evidence of left ventricular hypertrophy in a general aged population. Am J Cardiol 1994;74:385-90.
19. Shub C, Klein AS, Zachariah PK, Bailey KR, Tajik AJ. Determination of left ventricular mass by echocardiography in a normal population: effect of age and sex in addition to body size. Mayo Clin Proc 1994;69:205-11.
20. Ross J. Afterload mismatch in aortic and mitral valve disease: Implications for surgical therapy. J Am Coll Cardiol 1985;5:811-26.
21. Henry WL, Bonow RO, Borer JS et al. Evaluation of aortic valve replacement in patients with valvular aortic stenosis. Circulation 1980;61:814-25.
22. Schuler G, Peterson KL, Johnson AD. Serial noninvasive assessment of left ventricular hypertrophy and function after surgical correction of aortic regurgitation. Am J Cardiol 1979;44:585-94.
23. Gaasch WH, Carroll JD, Levine HJ, Criscitiello MG. Chronic aortic regurgitation: prognostic value of the left ventricular end-diastolic and the end-systolic dimension and end-diastolic radius/thickness ratio. J Am Coll Cardiol 1983;1:775-82.
24. Gaasch WH, Levine HJ, Zile MR. Chronic aortic and mitral regurgitation: mechanical consequences of the lesion and the results of surgical correction. In: Gaasch WH, Levine HJ, editors. The Ventricle. Boston: Martinus Nijhof Publishers; 1985; p. 237-58.
25. Carabello BA. Mitral valve disease. Curr Probl Cardiol 1993;18:421-80.
26. Eckberg DL, Gault JH, Bouchard RL, Karliner JS, Ross J. Jr. Mechanics of left ventricular contraction in

chronic severe mitral regurgitation. Circulation 1973;47:1252-9.

27. Wisenbaugh T, Spann JF, Carabello BA. Differences in myocardial performance and load between patients with similar amounts of chronic aortic versus chronic mitral regurgitation. J Am Coll Cardiol 1984;3:916-23.

28. Gaasch WH, Zile MR. Left ventricular function after surgical correction of chronic mitral regurgitation. Eur Heart J 1991 12 (suppl B):48-51.

29. Starling MR, Kirsh MM, Montgomery DG et al. Impaired left ventricular contractile function in patients with long-term mitral regurgitation and normal ejection fraction. J Am Coll Cardiol 1993;22:239-50.

30. Starling MR. Effects of valve surgery on left ventricular contractile function in patients with long-term mitral regurgitation. Circulation 1985;92:811-8.

31. Enriquez-Sarano M, Schaff HV, Orszulak TA et al. Congestive heart failure after surgical correction of mitral regurgitation: A long-term study. Circulation 1995;92:2496-503.

32. Quinones MA, Gaasch WH, Alexander JK. Influence of acute changes in preload, afterload contractile state and heart rate on ejection and isovolumic indices of myocardial contractility in man. Circulation 1976;53:293-302.

33. Wisenbaugh T. Does normal pump function belie muscle dysfunction in patients with chronic severe mitral regurgitation? Circulation 1988;77:515-25.

34. Kass DA, Maughan WL, Guo ZM, Kono A, Sunagawa K, Sagawa K. Comparative influence of load versus inotropic states on indexes of ventricular contractility:experimental and theoretical analysis based on P-V relationships. Circulation 1987;76:1422-36.

35. Schuler G, Peterson KL, Johnson AD et al. Temporal response of left ventricular performance to mitral valve surgery. Circulation 1979;59:1218-31.

36. Zile MR, Gaasch WH, Carroll JD, Levine HJ. Chronic mitral regurgitation: predictive value of preoperative echocardiographic indexes of left ventricular function and wall stress. J Am Coll Cardiol 1984;3:235-42.

37. David TE, Uden DE, Strauss HD. The importance of the mitral apparatus in left ventricular function after correction of mitral regurgitation. Circulation 1983;68:II-76-82.

38. Goldman ME, Mora F, Guarino T, Fuster V, Mindlich BP. Mitral valvuloplasty is superior to valve replacement for preservation of left ventricular function:An intra-operative two-dimensional echocardiographic study. J Am Coll Cardiol 1987;10:568-75.

12. MYOCARDIAL HYPERTROPHY AND FAILURE: A MOLECULAR APPROACH

J.M. van Dantzig, R. Bronsaer, P.A.F.M. Doevendans

Summary

Molecular biology is increasing our understanding of cardiomyocyte changes that occur during hypertrophy and its transition to heart failure. In the present chapter, an overview is presented regarding the way cardiomyocytes sense mechanical overload and the consequent changes in metabolism, cellular energy and myocardial calcium kinetics. Furthermore, an outline is presented of the application of murine animal models to investigate these molecular changes.

Introduction

The etiology of heart failure is gradually being determined. A genetic cause of familial cardiomyopathy has recently been identified and mutations in a splice site of the dystrophin gene were shown to cause X-linked cardiomyopathy.[1] Mutations in DNA coding for actin are related to autosomal dominantly inherited dilated cardiomyopathy.[2] In other families, loci have been determined but mutations are still to be identified. It is estimated that 20% of all cardiomyopathies have a genetic background. Also, dilated cardiomyopathy may be part of a more extensive syndrome, in which mutations in mitochondrial DNA are related to abnormalities in neurons and both skeletal and heart muscle.[3] Searches for genetic polymorphisms associated with an increased risk of cardiomyopathy have been conducted, without convincing evidence thus far.[4,5] In hypertensive heart disease and myocardial damage due to coronary artery disease, pump failure is preceded by myocardial hypertrophy. Knowledge of stimuli and mechanisms related to hypertrophy are therefore important, and insight into the transition from hypertrophy to failure may lead to strategies to prevent failure.[6,7] This chapter will address the molecular aspects of myocardial hypertrophy and failure.

E. E. van der Wall et al.(eds.), Left Ventricular Hypertrophy, 151-161.
© 1999 *Kluwer Academic Publishers. Printed in the Netherlands.*

Pathophysiology of hypertrophy

Hypertrophy will occur as a reaction to long-standing pressure and volume overload. In pressure overload, for instance due to hypertension or aortic valvular stenosis, myofibrils replicate in parallel and consequent widening of individual myocytes will thicken the myocardium. In volume overload in for instance valvular regurgitation or intracardiac shunts, serial replication of sarcomeres will lead to lengthening of individual myocytes. The increase in ventricular volume will induce increased wall tension. This will in turn stimulate myocardial thickening, which will normalize wall tension.[8] During the development of hypertrophy the synthesis of matrix proteins will increase. In addition, due to coronary vascular changes the subendocardial perfusion will decrease.[8]

Myocyte hypertrophy

Hypertrophy may be studied at the level of the individual myocyte by molecular techniques. For this purpose, cultured myocytes from neonatal rat hearts are used.[9]

In this model, hypertrophy can be induced in several ways, e.g. administration of catecholamines, angiotensin-II, endothelin, growth factors (e.g. Insulin like Growth Factor-I, cardiotrophin) and mechanical stretch.[10,11] The membrane receptors for these hormones are coupled to G-proteins, which through several intermediate phosphorylating reactions activate second messengers as protein-kinase C (PKC) en mitogen activated protein-kinase (MAP).[12] This will ultimately activate nuclear proteins, the so-called transcription factors, with consequent changes in gene expression.[7] These transcriptional changes at the transcriptional level induce expression of a fetal gene program, with among others re-expression of atrial natriuretic factor (ANF), skeletal alpha-actin, atrial myosin light chain (MLC-2a) and (in rats, but not in humans) β-myosin heavy chain (Table 1).[13] These genes are therefore used as molecular markers of hypertrophy.

The promoters of these genes - briefly, molecular switches that govern expression of the relevant gene - may be investigated after isolation by coupling promoter sequences to reporter genes. The reporter genes code for easily identifiable proteins, absent in normal cells. The luciferase gene, which makes fire-flies emit light, or the 'green fluorescent protein' may be used for this purpose.[14,15] The DNA construct of promoter and reporter gene is introduced (transfected) into cardiomyocytes. An example of such an experiment is shown in figure 1, displaying the effects of endothelin and phenylephrin on promoter activity of ANF and MLC-2a in ventricular myocytes.

Table 1. Changes in gene expression during hypertrophy.

Activated	Inactivated	Failure
Na$^+$\Ca^{2+} exchanger	Ca^{2+} channels (SERCA, L-type)	Cytokines (TNF-α)
Natriuretic factors	Phospholamban	?
Sarcomere genes (MLC-2a)	Potassium channel (Kv1.5)	
Growth factors (ET-1, IGF-1)		
Transcription factors		

SERCA: sarcoplasmatic reticulum Ca^{2+} ATP-ase; MLC-2a: atrial myosin light chain 2; ET-1: endothelin-1; IGF-1: insuline like growth factor 1; TNF-α: Tumor necrosis factor alfa.

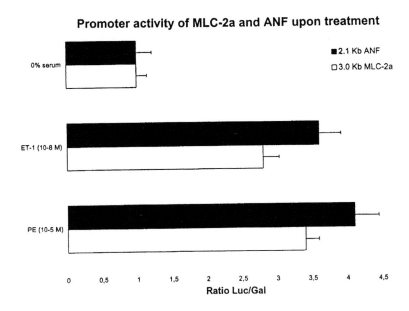

Figure 1. Results of a transfection experiment in neonatal rat ventricular myocytes with promoter fragments linked to the luciferase reporter gene. Cells are treated with endothelin or phenylephrin. Stimulation of the myocytes leads to activation of the promoter of the myosin light chain and atrial natriuretic factor gene.

These cells increase in size, in concert with activation of the promoters, as evidenced by an increased activity of the reporter gene (in this example, luciferase).

Note that the mentioned neurohormonal agonists not only cause hypertrophy *in vitro*, but are also activated in human heart failure. For many of these neurohormonal systems, activation has been related to worse prognosis. By inhibiting the angiotensin converting enzyme or by treatment with beta-adrenergic blocking drugs- the outlook of heart failure patients can be improved.[16,17] Such findings underline the close relation between myocardial hypertrophy and failure.

Mechanoreception

The mechanisms by which cardiomyocytes detect stretch are as yet imprecisely defined. *In vitro* experiments have revealed several potential mechanisms. Mechanically stretched cultured myocytes will develop a less differentiated fetal genotype. Deforming myocytes cultured on elastic membranes will induce release of angiotensin-II (AT-II), and increase MAP-kinase activity and protein synthesis. This hypertrophic response may be blocked by inhibition of the sodium/hydrogen exchanger (NHE).[18] NHE is activated following mechanical stretch by phosphorylation of the cytoplasmic domain, probably mediated by PKC.[19]

Stretching feline papillary muscle increased intracellular pH, which could be prevented by blocking NHE, or the angiotensin-1 receptor, endothelin receptors and PKC, respectively.[20] Stretch thus increases NHE activity, involving an auto-paracrine mechanism in which PKC, AT-II and endothelin play crucial roles.

The importance of mechanical load on cardiomyocytes in inducing and perpetuating heart failure in patients is suggested by the beneficial effect of prolonged circulatory unloading with mechanical assist devices.[21] Cardiomyocytes isolated from six patients showed decreased velocities of contraction and relaxation, with considerable improvements noted after mechanical support during a mean of 111 days.

Metabolic remodeling

Oxidation of fatty acids supplies two-thirds of the energy requirements of the normal heart, the remainder being supplied by carbohydrates such as glucose and glycogen.

Both in animal models and clinically, hypertrophy is associated with a shift from fatty acid to glucose utilization, concurrent with increased formation of lactate.[22,23] This suggests that not all myocardial energy demands are being met under these circumstances. The expression of genes related to fatty acid cellular uptake, cytosolic handling and mitochondrial oxidation is decreased in the hypertrophic heart.[24] Possibly, direct genomic effects of oxygen, carbohydrates and fatty acids on gene expression are involved, analogous to the mechanism through which renal hypoxia induces erythropoetin secretion.

Myocardial energy

Increased myocardial load is not paralleled by an increase in capillary density. The diminished capillary density will decrease delivery of oxygen and substrate to the mitochondrion and decreased levels of energy-rich compounds in hypertrophic and failing hearts have been demonstrated, in vivo.[25] The presence of energy-rich compounds can be measured by magnetic resonance spectroscopy.[26] In patients with mitral regurgitation, the ratio of phosphocreatine (PCr) to adenosinetriphosphate (ATP) is decreased in proportion to the severity of the regurgitation, as evidenced both by echocardiography (left ventricular internal dimensions, severity of regurgitation) and functional class.[27] The PCr/ATP ratio was found to be prognostically relevant in patients with heart failure due to dilated cardiomyopathy.[28] This is related to decreased activity of creatin kinase (CK), the enzyme which catalyzes the transfer of phosphate form PCr to ATP.[29] Energy stored in PCr may be considered as reserve to cope with hemodynamic or metabolic overload. Inhibition of CK impedes use of these energy stores, with consequently decreased contractile reserve as shown in animal experiments.[30] In failing hearts, CK-activity is clearly decreased, both in animals and in humans.[31,32] In the normal heart, this is compensated for by glycolysis and oxydative phosphorylation, and presumably, these mechanisms are exhausted in failing hearts.

Myocardial calcium kinetics

Important changes in myocardial handling of calcium, the ion coupling electrical excitation to mechanical contraction, occur in hypertrophy and failure. Four proteins are relevant in this respect.[33] The ryanodin receptor, localized on the junctional sarcoplasmic reticulum (SR), is the channel allowing release of calcium form the SR to the sarcolemma, thus inducing contraction. The sarcoplasmic calcium ATP-ase (SERCA) actively promotes relaxation by pumping calcium from the sarcolemma to the sarcoplasmic reticulum. This pump is modulated by phospholamban. Phosphorylation of phospholamban, e.g. after β-adrenergic stimulation, importantly increases SERCA activity. Calcium is stored in the sarcoplasmic reticulum bound to proteins (calsequestrin, calreticulin). Extracellular calcium may flow into the sarcolemma through the dihydropyridin receptor (L-type calcium channel).

In animal models of hypertrophy and failure induced by pressure overload (e.g. aortic banding) decreased SERCA expression both at the transcriptional level (decreased m-RNA) and protein level have been demonstrated. The functional relevance of lower SERCA levels was supported by a decreased velocity of relaxation.[34,35] SERCA decreases proportional to the level of hypertrophy, indicating that for this protein there is no qualitative but rather a quantitative difference between hypertrophy and failure.

In animal experiments of tachycardia-induced heart failure and in explanted hearts from transplant recipients, the peak tension of contraction is decreased, as are the velocities of contraction and relaxation.[36,37]

By use of aeqorin, which emits light when bound to calcium, calcium fluxes during contraction and relaxation were shown to be slowed in myocytes isolated from human failing hearts, and total calcium inflow is decreased.[37,38] Also in isolated myocytes, these changes were shown to be related to decreased SERCA expression.[39,40] Parallel changes of phospholamban and ryanodin receptor occur, but the expression of calsequestrin is unchanged in heart failure.[41]

Murine models

More recently, genetically modified mice have been applied to study hypertrophy and failure. The small size and high heart rate of these experimental animals pose technical challenges in measuring functional parameters by invasive hemodynamic investigation, two-dimensional and Doppler-echocardiography and magnetic resonance imaging (MRI).

However, the ease of genetic modification and the short reproductive cycle allow unique opportunities to investigate functional consequences of genetic changes.[42]

Genetic manipulation consists of either overexpression (more protein, transgenesis) or decreased expression ('knock-out', less protein) of the investigated gene. For instance, to study the relevance of increased levels of expression tumor necrosis factor-α in myocardium of patients with heart failure, this gene was expressed in mouse hearts.[43,44] This resulted in mortality from heart failure, cardiomegaly and hypertrophy, decreased systolic function as evidenced by MRI, decreased isoprenalin-induced dP/dt rise as well as ANF expression in the ventricular myocardium.

More germane to the question of hypertrophy and failure was an experiment in which the gene coding for Gα-q protein was overexpressed.[45] As stated, receptor dependent activation of G proteins is closely associated with induction of hypertrophy. Myocytes of these mice showed decreased contractility and they expressed a fetal gene program. Only after surgical aortic banding did myocardial weight increase in both groups. The pattern of hypertrophy was strikingly different, with the Gα-q transgenic mice demonstrating increased ventricular dimensions with unchanged wall thickness (eccentric hypertrophy), while animals in the control group had unchanged ventricular size with markedly increased wall thickness (concentric hypertrophy). In Gα-q mice, hypertrophy was associated with striking systolic dysfunction. Thus a single gene may modify susceptibility for heart failure resulting from an hemodynamic intervention. The authors point out that the concept of the transition of compensated hypertrophy to decompensated heart failure may not be correct. Rather, hemodynamic loading may induce a cardiomyopathy of overload, in which maintained function is irrevocably associated with deleterious changes in the composition of contractile proteins induced by fetal gene expression, mediated by among others Gα-q stimulation. Such changes may decrease the ability to handle further hemodynamic loading, as in this experiment.

Hypertrophy to failure

Dilatation without previous wall thickening is prominent in toxic and infectious cardiomyopathies in man.[46-48] The rapidity with which disease develops and myocardial reserve determine the possibility of a hypertrophic response, with a possible role for genetic predisposition. In general, hypertension and ischemic heart disease will in first instance cause increased wall thickness, with consequent diastolic heart failure. The latter is also prominent in hypertrophic cardiomyopathy.[49]

Why and how hypertrophy progresses to failure is at present not fully explained. Continued exposure to hemodynamic, ischemic, neurohumoral and cytokine stimulation may not only alter gene expression but also induce cell death. The latter may occur through either necrosis or apoptosis, where apoptosis signifies programmed cell death without inflammation. Recent findings in humans suggest a role for apoptosis in myocardial remodeling, both after myocardial infarction and in end-stage heart failure.[50,51]

It is unclear whether transition from hypertrophy to failure is determined by activation of a specific, as yet unknown, gene program, or whether cardiac function deteriorates as a consequence of the preceding defined hypertrophic gene expression (Figure 2).[52] Possibly, the relative contribution to the development of heart failure of such qualitative as opposed to quantitative genetic changes differ in relation to the primary myocardial insult.

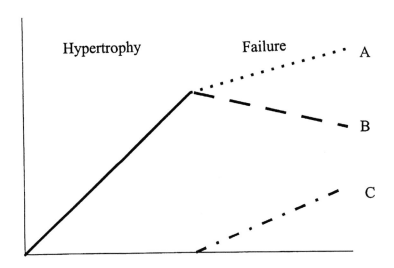

Figure 2. Hypothesis with regard to the pattern of gene expression during hypertrophy and failure. Hypertrophy is characterized by fetal gene expression (extended line). Situation A: Gradual transition from hypertrophy to failure. B: Failure is characterized by a decrease in expression of the compensating genes. C: Start of a specific gene expression program during failure.

Conclusion

Non-physiologic myocardial hypertrophy appears to jeopardize cardiac function. Efforts at detecting, preventing and treating hypertrophy therefore appear of paramount importance.

References

1. Milasin J, Muntoni F, Severini GM, et al. A point mutation in the 5' splice site of the dystrophin gene first intron responsible for X-linked dilated cardiomyopathy. Hum Mol Genet 1996;5:73-9.

2. Olson TM, Michels VV, Thibodeau SN, Tai YS, Keating MT. Actin mutations in dilated cardiomyopathy, a heritable form of heart failure. Science 1998;280:750-2.

3. Doevendans PA, Van Dantzig J, Meijer H, Schaap C. Molecular genetics of human cardiomyopathies. In: Peters RJG, Piek JJ, editors. Molecular cardiology in clinical perspective. Amsterdam: Knoll; 1997: p. 33-53.

4. Kubota T, McNamara DM, Wang JJ, et al. Effects of tumor necrosis factor gene polymorphisms on patients with congestive heart failure. VEST Investigators for TNF Genotype Analysis. Vesnarinone Survival Trial. Circulation 1998;97:2499-501.

5. Yamada Y, Ichihara S, Fujimura T, Yokota M. Lack of association of polymorphisms of the angiotensin converting enzyme and angiotensinogen genes with nonfamilial hypertrophic or dilated cardiomyopathy. Am J Hypertens 1997;10:921-8.

6. Doevendans PA, Reneman RS, Van Bilsen M, editors. Cardiovascular specific gene expression. Dordrecht: Kluwer; 1999.

7. Doevendans PA, Van Gilst WH, Laarse A, Van Bilsen M. Molecular cardiology part I: Gene transcription in the cardiovascular system. Cardiologie 1997;4:221-9.

8. Van der Laarse A, Ruwhof C, Van Wamel JET, Van Gilst WH, Doevendans PA, Van Bilsen M. Molecular cardiology. Part 2: Molecular aspects of cardiac hypertrophy and heart failure. Cardiologie 1997;4:328-33.

9. Simpson P, Shoshana S. Differentiation of rat myocytes in single cultures with and without proliferating non-myocardial cells. Circ Res 1982;50:101-16.

10. Ross JJ, Hongo M. The role of hypertrophy and growth factors in heart failure. J Card Fail 1996;2:S121-S128

11. Wollert KC, Taga T, Saito M, et al. Cardiotrophin-1 activates a distinct form of cardiac muscle cell hypertrophy. Assembly of sarcomeric units in series VIA gp130/leukemia inhibitory factor receptor-dependent pathways. J Biol Chem 1996;271:9535-45.

12. Thorburn J, Carlson M, Mansour SJ, Chien KR, Ahn NG, Thorburn A. Inhibition of a signaling pathway in cardiac muscle cells by active mitogen-activated protein kinase kinase. Mol Biol Cell 1995;6:1479-90.

13. Doevendans PA, Bronsaer R, Ruiz-Lozano P, Van Dantzig JM, Van Bilsen M. Expression of the atrial regulatory myosin light chain gene in ventriular cardiomyocytes. In: Doevendans PA, Reneman RS, Van Bilsen M, editors. Cardiovacular specific gene expression. Dordrecht: Kluwer; 1999.

14. Doevendans PA, Becker DA, An R, Kass RS. The utility of fluorescent *in vivo* reporter genes in molecular cardiology. Biochem Biophys Res Comm 1996;222:352-8.

15. Doevendans PA. Cardiac specific gene expression of the regulatory myosin light chains [PhD Thesis]. Maastricht: University of Maastricht, 1997.

16. Effects of enalapril on mortality in severe congestive heart failure. Results of the Cooperative North Scandinavian Enalapril Survival Study (CONSENSUS). The CONSENSUS Trial Study Group. N Engl J Med 1987;316:1429-35.

17. Heidenreich PA, Lee TT, Massie BM. Effect of beta-blockade on mortality in patients with heart failure: a meta-analysis of randomized clinical trials. J Am Coll Cardiol 1997;30:27-34.

18. Yamazaki T, Komuro I, Kudoh S, et al. Role of ion channels and exchangers in mechanical stretch-induced cardiomyocyte hypertrophy. Circ Res 1998;82:430-7.

19. Sardet C, Franchi A, Pouyssegur J. Molecular cloning, primary structure, and expression of the human growth factor-activatable Na+/H+ antiporter. Cell 1989;56:271-80.

20. Cingolani HE, Alvarez BV, Ennis IL and Camilion de Hurtado MC. Stretch-induced alkalinization of feline papillary muscle. Circ Res 1998; 83:775-80.

21. Dipla K, Matiello JA, Jeevanandam V, Houser SR, Margulies KB. Myocyte recovery after mechanical circulatory support in humans with end-stage heart failure. Circulation 1998;97:2316-22.

22. Kagaya Y, Kanno Y, Takeyama D, et al. Effects of long-term pressure overload on regional myocardial glucose and free fatty acid uptake in rats. A quantitative autoradiographic study. Circulation 1990;81:1353-61.

23. Tadamura E, Kudoh T, Hattori N, et al. Impairment of BMIPP uptake precedes abnormalities in oxygen and glucose metabolism in hypertrophic cardiomyopathy. J Nucl Med 1998;39:390-6.

24. Sack MN, Rader TA, Park S, Bastin J, McCune SA, Kelly DP. Fatty acid oxidation enzyme gene expression is downregulated in the failing heart. Circulation 1996;94:2837-42.

25. Ebert BL, Gleadle JM, O'Rourke JF, Bartlett SM, Poulton J, Ratcliffe PJ. Isoenzyme-specific regulation of genes involved in energy metabolism by hypoxia: similarities with the regulation of erythropoietin. Biochem J 1996;313:809-14.

26. De Roos A, Doornbos J, Luyten PR, Oosterwaal LJ, Van der Wall EE, den Hollander J. Cardiac metabolism in patients with dilated and hypertrophic cardiomyopathy: assessment with proton-decoupled P-31 MR spectroscopy. J Magn Reson Imaging 1992;2:711-9.

27. Conway MA, Bottomley PA, Ouwerkerk R, Radda GK, Rajagopalan B. Mitral regurgitation: impaired systolic function, eccentric hypertrophy, and increased severity are linked to lower phosphocreatine/ATP ratios in humans. Circulation 1998;97:1716-23.

28. Neubauer S, Horn M, Cramer M, et al. Myocardial phosphocreatine-to-ATP ratio is a predictor of mortality in patients with dilated cardiomyopathy. Circulation 1997;96:2190-6.

29. Ingwall JS. ATP synthesis in the normal and failing heart. In: Poole-Wilson PA, et al. editors. Heart failure. New York: Churchill Livingstone; 1997. p. 75-85.

30. Van Deursen J, Heerschap A, Oerlemans F, et al. Skeletal muscles of mice deficient in muscle creatine kinase lack burst activity. Cell 1993;74:621-31.

31. Neubauer S, Horn M, Naumann A, et al. Impairment of energy metabolism in intact residual myocardium of rat hearts with chronic myocardial infarction. J Clin Invest 1995;95:1092-100.

32. Van der Laarse A, Hollaar L, Kok SW, et al. Myocardial creatine kinase-MB concentration in normal and explanted human hearts and released from hearts of patients with acute myocardial infarction. Clin Physiol Biochem 1992;9:11-7.

33. Arai M, Matsui H, Periasamy M. Sarcoplasmic reticulum gene expression in cardiac hypertrophy and heart failure. Circ Res 1994;74:555-64.

34. Schouten VJ, Vliegen HW, Van der Laarse A, Huysmans HA. Altered calcium handling at normal contractility in hypertrophied rat heart. J Mol Cell Cardiol 1990;22:987-98.

35. Bastie DD, Levitsky D, Rappaport L, et al. Function of the sarcoplasmic reticulum and expression of its Ca2(+)-ATPase gene in pressure overload-induced cardiac hypertrophy in the rat. Circ Res 1990;66:554-64.

36. Perreault CL, Shannon RP, Komamura K, Vatner SF, Morgan JP. Abnormalities in intracellular calcium regulation and contractile function in myocardium from dogs with pacing-induced heart failure. J Clin Invest 1992;89:932-8.

37. Gwathmey JK, Copelas L, MacKinnon R, et al. Abnormal intracellular calcium handling in myocardium from patients with end-stage heart failure. Circ Res 1987;61:70-6.

38. Morgan JP, Erny RE, Allen PD, Grossman W, Gwathmey JK. Abnormal intracellular calcium handling, a major cause of systolic and diastolic dysfunction in ventricular myocardium from patients with heart failure. Circulation 1990;81 part III:III21-III32

39. Mercadier JJ, Lompre AM, Duc P, et al. Altered sarcoplasmic reticulum Ca2(+)-ATPase gene expression in the human ventricle during end-stage heart failure. J Clin Invest 1990;85:305-9.

40. Arai M, Alpert NR, MacLennan DH, Barton P, Periasamy M. Alterations in sarcoplasmic reticulum gene expression in human heart failure. A possible mechanism for alterations in systolic and diastolic properties of the failing myocardium. Circ Res 1993;72:463-9.

41. Takahashi T, Allen PD, Lacro RV. Expression of dihydropyridine receptor Ca^{2+} channel and calsequestrin genes in the myocardium of patients with end-stage heart failure. J Clin Invest 1992;90:1713-9.

42. Doevendans PA, Daemen M, de Muinck E, Smits J. Cardiovascular phenotyping in mice. Cardiovas Res 1998;39:34-49.

43. Kubota T, McTiernan CF, Frye CS, et al. Dilated cardiomyopathy in transgenic mice with cardiac- specific overexpression of tumor necrosis factor-alpha. Circ Res 1997;81:627-35.

44. Bryant D, Becker L, Richardson J, et al. Cardiac failure in transgenic mice with myocardial expression of tumor necrosis factor-alpha. Circulation 1998;97:1375-81.

45. Sakata Y, Hoit BD, Liggett SB, Walsh RA, Dorn GW. Decompensation of pressure-overload hypertrophy in G alpha q-overexpressing mice. Circulation 1998;97:1488-95.

46. McKenna CJ, Codd MB, McCann HA, Sugrue DD. Alcohol consumption and idiopathic dilated cardiomyopathy: a case control study. Am Heart J 1998;135:833-7.

47. Singal PK, Iliskovic N. Doxorubicin-induced cardiomyopathy. N Engl J Med 1998;339:900-5.

48. Barbaro G, Di Lorenzo G, Grisorio B, Barbarini G. Incidence of dilated cardiomyopathy and detection of HIV in myocardial cells of HIV-positive patients. Gruppo Italiano per lo Studio Cardiologico dei Pazienti Affetti da AIDS. N Engl J Med 1998;339:1093-9.

49. Van der Wall E. Hypertrophic cardiomyopathy. Morphology, pathophysiology and clinical implications. Neth J Cardiol 1988;1:91-103.

50. Saraste A, Pulkki K, Kallajoki M, et al. Apotosis in human acute myocardial infarction Circulation 1997;95:320-3.

51. Narula J, Haider N, Virmani R, et al. Apoptosis in myocytes in end-stage heart failure. N Engl J Med 1996;335:1182-9.

52. Lorell BH. Transition from hypertrophy to failure. Circulation 1997;96:3824-7.

13. HYPERTROPHY: CLINICAL RELEVANCE OF GENOTYPE

EINTHOVEN LECTURE 1999

K. SCHWARTZ

Summary

In recent years, molecular genetic studies in humans have shown that abnormal cardiac growth can result from molecular alterations within the myocardium, unrelated to changes in afterload. In humans, mutations in genes encoding components of the contractile apparatus of the cardiac myocyte produce familial hypertrophic cardiomyopathy (FHC). FHC is genetically heterogeneous and all the known disease genes encode sarcomeric proteins: β-myosin heavy chain, cardiac troponin T, α-tropomyosin, cardiac myosin binding protein C, essential and regulatory myosin light chains and cardiac troponin I. There is also a striking allelic heterogeneity, and more than 100 mutations were found so far. The two major genes are those encoding β-myosin heavy chain (MYH7) and cardiac myosin binding protein C (MYBPC3). The clinical relevance of these observations will be discussed.

Introduction

In recent years, molecular genetic studies in humans as well as the capacity to selectively mutate genes or create excessive or deleted gene expression in muscle have shown that abnormal cardiac growth can result from molecular alterations within the myocardium, unrelated to changes in afterload. In humans, mutations in genes encoding components of the contractile apparatus of the cardiac myocyte produce hypertrophic cardiomyopathy. It is a complex cardiac disease with unique pathophysiological characteristics and a great diversity of morphologic, functional and clinical features.[1,2] Although hypertrophic cardiomyopathy has been regarded largely as a relatively uncommon cardiac disease, the prevalence of echocardiographically defined hypertrophic cardiomyopathy in a large cohort

E. E. van der Wall et al.(eds.), Left Ventricular Hypertrophy, 163-174.

of apparently healthy young adults selected from a community-based general population was reported three years ago to be as high as 0.2%.[3] Familial disease with autosomal dominant inheritance predominates and is usually referred to as familial hypertrophic cardiomyopathy (FHC).

FHC is characterized by left and/or right ventricular hypertrophy, which is usually asymmetric and which can affect different regions of the ventricle. The interventricular septum is most commonly affected, with or without involvement of either the anterior wall or the posterior wall in continuity. A particular form of regional involvement affects the apex but spares the upper portion of the septum (apical hypertrophy).[1] Typically, the left ventricular volume is normal or reduced. Systolic gradients are common. Typical morphological changes include myocyte hypertrophy and disarray surrounding the areas of increased loose connective tissue. Patients with hypertrophic cardiomyopathy frequently report a reduced exercise capacity and functional limitation. Although the pathophysiological features of the disease that contribute to this limitation are complex and not fully understood, left ventricular outflow tract obstruction if present, is believed to contribute to increased filling pressures and a failure to augment cardiac output during exercise, leading to exertional symptoms. Arrhythmias and premature sudden deaths are common.[2, 3]

Disease genes for FHC

The first gene for FHC was mapped to chromosome 14q11.2-q12 using genome-wide linkage analysis in a large Canadian family.[4] Soon afterwards, FHC locus heterogeneity was subsequently reported[5,6] and confirmed by the mapping of the second FHC locus to chromosome 1q3 and of the third locus to chromosome 15q2.[7, 8] Carrier et al.[9] mapped the fourth FHC locus to chromosome 11p11.2. Four other loci were subsequently reported, located on chromosomes 7q3,[10] 3p21.2-3p21.3,[11] 12q23-q24.3[11] and 19p13.2-q13.2.[12] Several other families are not linked to any known FHC loci, indicating the existence of additional LQTS-causing genes.

All the disease genes encode proteins that are part of the sarcomere which is a complex structure with an exact stoichiometry and multiple sites of protein-protein interactions (Table 1, Figure 1 and review in[13]): three myofilament proteins, the β-myosin heavy chain (β-MyHC), the ventricular myosin essential light chain 1 (MLC-1s/v) and the ventricular myosin regulatory light chain 2 (MLC-2s/v); three thin filament proteins, cardiac troponin T (cTnT), cardiac troponin I (cTnI), and α-tropomyosin (α-TM); and finally one myosin-binding protein, the cardiac myosin binding protein C (cMyBP-C). Each of these proteins is encoded by multigene families which exhibit tissue specific, developmental, and physiologically regulated patterns of expression.

Table 1. FHC loci an disease genes.

Locus	Gene	Protein
14q11-12	MYH7	β-myosin heavy chain
1q3	TNNT2	Cardiac troponin T
15q2	TPM1	α-tropomyosin
11p11.2	MYBPC3	Cardiac myosin binding protein C
12q23q24.3	MYL2	Cardiac myosin regulatory light chain
3p	MYL3	Cardiac myosin essential light chain
19p13.2-q13.2	TNNC1	Cardiac troponin I
7q3	?	?

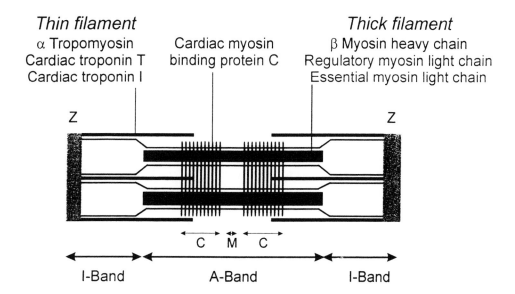

Figure 1. Schematic organization of the sarcomeric proteins associated with FHC. Reprinted with permission from the American Heart Association. Bonne G, Carrier L, Richard P, Hainque B, Schwartz K. Familial hypertrophic cardiomyopathy from mutations to functional defects. Circ Res 1998; 83:580-93.

Thick filament proteins

Myosin subunits

Myosin is the molecular motor that transduces energy from the hydrolysis of ATP into directed movement and that, by doing so, drives sarcomere shortening and muscle contraction. Cardiac myosin consists of two heavy chains (MyHC) and two pairs of light chains (MLC), referred to as essential (or alkali) light chains (MLC-1) and regulatory (or phosphorylatable) light chains (MLC-2), respectively. The myosin molecule is highly asymmetric, consisting of two globular heads joined to a long rod-like tail. The light chains are arranged in tandem in the head-tail junction. Their function is not fully understood. Neither myosin light chain type is required for the adenosine triphosphatase activity of the myosin head, but they probably modulate it in presence of actin and contribute to the rigidity of the neck which is hypothesized to function as a lever arm for generating an effective power stroke. Mutations were found in the heavy chains and in the two types of ventricular light chains (review in[13]).

Concerning the heavy chains, the β isoform (β-MyHC) is the major isoform of the human ventricle and of slow-twitch skeletal fibers. It is encoded by MYH7. At least 50 mutations were found in unrelated families with FHC (Table 2), and three hot spots for mutations were identified, codons 403, 719 and 741. All but three of these mutations are missense mutations located either in the head or in the head-rod junction of the molecule. The three exceptions are two 3 bp deletions that do not disrupt the reading frame, and a 2.4 kb deletion in the 3' region. In the kindred with the latter mutation, only the proband had developed clinically diagnosed hypertrophic cardiomyopathy at a very late onset (age, 59 years).

As for the light chains, the isoforms expressed in the ventricular myocardium and in the slow-twitch muscles are the so-called ventricular myosin regulatory light chains (MLC-2 s/v) encoded by MYL2, and the ventricular myosin essential light chain (MLC-1s/v) encoded by MYL3. They both belong to the superfamily of EF-hand proteins. Two missense mutations were found in MYL3, and five in MYL2 (Table 2).

Table 2. FHC mutations.

MYH7		MYL2	MYL3	MYBPC3		TNNT2		TNNI3		TPM1
Missense mutations	Other mutations	Missense mutations	Missense mutations	Missense mutations	Truncation mutations	Missense mutations	Other mutations	Missense mutations	Other mutations	Missense mutations
A26V	delG10	A13T	V149M	E258K	D1g-a	189N	delE170	R145Q	delK183	A63V
V591	**delE930**	**F18L**	H154R	E451Q	**D5g-a**	R102W	D1	R145G		K70T
T1241	delG1931-	E22K		R495Q	A-2a-g	R102Q		R162W		D175N
R143Q	E1935	**R58Q**		R502Q	E451Q	**R102L**		G203S		E180G
Y162C		P95A		**E542Q**	**E542q**	A114V		K206Q		
N187K				E654H	Δ1-593	F120I				
Q222K				**N755K**	**A-2a-g**	E173K				
N232S					Δ1-698	E254D				
F244L					**D1g-a**	R288C				
K246Q					D1g-t					
R249Q					**BPa-g**					
G256E					I1-791					
A259E					**Δ5-845**					
I263T					Δ2-955					
M349T					Q969+					
K383N					D1g-a					
R403Q					I2-1042					
R403W					D5g-c					
R403L					D1g-a					
R453C					D1g-a					
E483LF					**X12/Δ4-1220**					
513C					X18-1254					
G584R										
D587V										
N602S										
V606M										
K615N										
G716R										
R719W										
R719Q										
R719W										
R723C										
P731L										
I736M										
G741R										
G741R										
G741W										
D778G										
S782N										
A797T										
R870H										
L908V										
E924K										
E930K										
E935K										
E949K										
E1205K										

Animo acids are named according to the usual genetic code. Bold characters indicate the mutations found withint the French INSERM collborative network.

Myosin binding protein C (MyBP-C)

MyBP-C is located in the sarcomere A band. Its function is uncertain, but, for a decade, evidence has existed to indicate both structural and regulatory roles. Partial extraction of cMyBP-C from rat skinned cardiac myocytes and rabbit skeletal muscle fibers alters Ca^{2+}-sensitive tension,[14] and it was shown that phosphorylation of cMyBP-C alters myosin cross-bridges in native thick filaments, suggesting that cMyBP-C can modify force production in activated cardiac muscles.

The cardiac isoform is encoded by the MYBPC3 gene. We have recently determined its organization and sequence.[15] Gautel et al.[16] showed that three distinct regions are specific to the cardiac isoform: the NH_2-terminal domain C0 Ig-I containing 101 residues, the MyBP-C motif (a 105-residue stretch linking the C1 and C2 Ig-I domains), and a 28-residue loop inserted in the C5 Ig-I domain. We and others recently showed that cMyBP-C is specifically expressed in the heart during human and murine development.[17, 18]

Thirty MYBPC3 mutations were found in unrelated families with FHC (Table 2). Twenty of them result in aberrant transcripts that are predicted to encode COOH-terminal truncated cardiac MyBP-C polypeptides lacking at least the myosin-binding domain. Seven others result in mutated or deleted proteins without disruption of the reading frame: five are missense mutations, one is a splice donor site mutation in intron 27, and one is a 18-residue duplication in exon 33. Finally, three mutations are predicted to produce either a mutated protein or a truncated one: two are missense mutations in exon 15 and 17 and one is a branch point mutation in intron 23.

Thin filament proteins

The troponin complex and tropomyosin constitute the Ca^{2+}-sensitive switch that regulates the contraction of cardiac muscle fibers. Mutations were found in the α-TM and in two of the subunits of the troponin complex: cTnI, the inhibitory subunit, and cTnT, the tropomyosin-binding subunit.

α-TM is encoded by TPM1. The cardiac isoform is expressed both in the ventricular myocardium and in fast twitch skeletal muscles. It shares the overall structure of other tropomyosins that are rod-like proteins that possess a simple dimeric α-coiled-coil structure in parallel orientation along their entire length. Four missense mutations were found in unrelated FHC families (Table 2). Two of them, A63V and K70T, are located in exon 2b within the consensus pattern of sequence repeats of α-TM and could alter tropomyosin binding to actin. Mutations D175N and E180G are both located within constitutive exon 5, in a region near the calcium-dependent TnT binding domain.

cTnT is encoded by TNNT2. In human cardiac muscle, multiple isoforms of cTnT have been described which are expressed in the fetal, adult and diseased heart, and which result from alternative splicing of the single gene TNNT2.[19, 20] The precise physiological relevance of these isoforms is currently poorly understood. We have partially established the organization of the human gene, and this allows us now to precisely identify the position of the mutations within exons, including those alternatively spliced during development, and also to use an amino acid numbering that reflects the full coding potential of human TNNT2.[21, 22] Eleven mutations were found in unrelated FHC families, three of which are located in a hot spot (codon 102) (Table 2). Ten mutations are missense ones located between exons 9 and 17, one mutation is a 3 bp deletion located in exon 12 that does not disrupt the coding frame, and the last is located in the intron 16 splice donor site and is predicted to produce a truncated protein in which the C-terminal binding sites are disrupted.

cTnI is encoded by TNNI3. The cTnI isoform is expressed only in cardiac muscles. Cooperative binding of cTnI to actin-tropomyosin is a unique property of the cardiac variant. Six mutations were recently identified (Table 2). Five are missense mutations located in exons 7 and 8, and one is a K183D mutation that does not disrupt the coding frame.

How mutations in sarcomeric genes cause FHC

Any consideration of the molecular mechanisms by which mutations cause FHC must be consistent with the dominant mode of disease inheritance. Most mutations found in the MYH7, MYL3, MYL2, TPM1, TNNT2 and TNNI3 genes are missense ones or small deletions without frameshift that are predicted to lead to mutant proteins, whereas most of those found in the MYBPC3 gene are splicing consensus sites, deletions, insertions or nonsense mutations that are predicted to lead to truncated proteins. Mutant proteins are presumably present in the tissue and act in a dominant fashion probably as poison polypeptides, i.e. they are incorporated in the sarcomere and change the function of the wild type protein and/or the assembly of the sarcomeric filaments. The incorporation of mutant protein in vivo has been demonstrated for two mutations, the R403Q MYH7 and the D175N TPM1 mutation. This poison polypeptide hypothesis is also supported by a variety of results obtained in vitro and by findings in nematodes in which missense mutations produce stable polypeptides that are incorporated into myofibrils and disrupt the sarcomere assembly.

The situation is more complex when mutations leading to truncated proteins are involved. The mutations could induce «null alleles» potentially leading to haploinsufficiency: the production of insufficient quantities of a normal sarcomeric protein would produce an imbalance in the stoichiometry of the thick- or the thin-filament components that would be sufficient to alter the sarcomeric structure and function. In this case, the null alleles would exhibit a dominant phenotype. This is what occurs in heterozygous mice for a-MHC null alleles that have severe impairment of both contractility and relaxation.[23] None of the available data in FHC are however consistent with a mechanism of haploinsufficiency. A nonsense mutation has been found in the MYH7 gene that is predicted to encode a short variant of β-MHC protein (53-residues) in two healthy individuals (38 and 70 year-old).[24] This indicates that the single normal human cardiac MYH7 allele is sufficient to compensate for the heterozygous defect of the null allele. Two other recent studies addressed the «null allele» hypothesis, one by expressing truncated human cTnT in quail myotubes,[25] and the other by characterizing the transcripts and proteins present in an endomyocardial biopsy of a patient with a cMyBP-C splice donor site mutation.[26] None of the results were consistent with a mechanism of haploinsufficiency. It is clear that more studies are necessary to understand the molecular mechanisms by which mutations predicted to lead to truncated proteins cause FHC.

Genotype/phenotype relation in FHC

The pattern and extent of left ventricular hypertrophy in patients with hypertrophic cardiomyopathy vary greatly even in first-degree relatives and a high incidence of sudden deaths is reported in selected families. An important issue therefore is to determine whether the genotype heterogeneity observed in FHC accounts for the phenotypic diversity of the disease. However, the results must be seen as preliminary, because the available data relate to only a few hundred individuals, and it is obvious that although a given phenotype may be apparent in a small family, examining large or multiple families with the same mutation is required before drawing unambiguous conclusions. Several concepts nevertheless begin to emerge, at least for mutations in the MYH7, TNNT2 and MYBPC3 genes. For MYH7, it is clear that prognosis for patients with different mutations varies considerably (review in[27]). For example, the R403Q mutation appears to be associated with markedly reduced survival, whereas some others, such as the V606M one, appear more benign. The disease caused by TNNT2 mutations is usually associated with a 20% incidence of non-penetrance, a relatively mild and sometimes subclinical hypertrophy but a high incidence of sudden death which can occur even in the absence of significant clinical left ventricular hypertrophy.[7,28,29] In one family with a TNNT2 mutation, however, penetrance is complete, echocardiographic data show a wide range of hypertrophy and there was no sudden cardiac death.[21] Mutations in MYBPC3 seem to be characterized by specific clinical features with a mild phenotype in young subjects, a delayed age at the onset of symptoms and a favorable prognosis before the age of 40.[30-33]

Genetic studies have also revealed the presence of clinically healthy individuals carrying the mutant allele, which is associated in first-degree relatives with a typical phenotype of the disease. Several mechanisms could account for the large variability of the phenotypic expression of the mutations: the role of environmental differences and acquired traits (e.g., differences in lifestyle, risk factors, and exercise) and finally the existence of modifier genes and/or polymorphisms that could modulate the phenotypic expression of the disease. The only significant results obtained so far concern the influence of the angiotensin-I converting enzyme insertion/deletion (ACE I/D) polymorphism. Association studies showed that, compared to a control population, the D allele is more common in patients with hypertrophic cardiomyopathy and in patients with a high incidence of sudden cardiac death.[34, 35] We recently showed that the association between the D allele and hypertrophy is observed in the case of MYH7 R403 codon mutations, but not with MYBPC3 mutation carriers,[36] raising the concept of multiple genetic modifiers in FHC.

Conclusions

Although we have only begun to dissect the molecular mechanisms leading to FHC, mutations in sarcomeric genes are now recognized as a principal cause of this disease. This offers promising perspectives for clinicians: revisiting diagnosis criteria, prognosis stratification and identification of healthy carriers. Clearly, more studies that would improve our understanding of the relation between phenotype and genotype are warranted, and the ultimate value of genotyping in FHC may be primarily to define an "at-risk" group. This is an area that deserves further careful clinical research.

The present focus on sarcomeric proteins should not, however, preclude the search of other genetic origins: the finding that both hypertrophic and dilated cardiomyopathies in hamster are caused by mutations in the *-sarcoglycan gene encoding a protein of the dystrophin-associated glycoprotein complex[37] could provide significant new insights into the pathogenesis of hypertrophic cardiomyopathy in man. Conversely, it was recently reported that mutations in another sarcomeric gene, cardiac actin, cause dilated cardiomyopathy in humans.[38] These two sets of data raise the important issue whether hypertrophic and dilated cardiomyopathies are inherently independent diseases or whether dilation is part of the FHC spectrum.

Acknowledgements

I would like to thank Stephanie Tardy for help in preparing this manuscript.

References

1. Wigle ED, Sasson Z, Henderson MA, et al. Hypertrophic cardiomyopathy. The importance of the site and the extent of hypertrophy. A review. Prog Cardiovasc Dis 1985;28:1-83.
2. Maron BJ, Bonow RO, Cannon RO, Leon MB, Epstein SE. Hypertrophic cardiomyopathy: interrelations of clinical manifestations, pathophysiology, and therapy. N Engl J Med 1987;316:780-9; and 844-52.
3. Maron BJ, Gardin JM, Flack JM, Gidding SS, Kurosaki TT, Bild DE. Prevalence of hypertrophic cardiomyopathy in a general population of young adults: echocardiographic analysis of 4111 subjects in the CARDIA study. Circulation 1995;92:785-9.
4. Jarcho JA, McKenna W, Pare JAP, et al. Mapping a gene for familial hypertrophic cardiomyopathy to chromosome 14q1. N Engl J Med. 1989;321:1372-8.
5. Solomon SD, Jarcho JA, Mc Kenna WJ, et al. Familial hypertrophic cardiomyopathy is a genetically heterogeneous disease. J Clin Invest. 1990; 86:993-9.
6. Schwartz K, Dufour C, Fougerousse F, et al. Exclusion of myosin heavy chain and cardiac actin gene involvement in hypertrophic cardiomyopathies of several French families. Circ Res. 1992; 71:3-8.
7. Watkins H, MacRae C, Thierfelder L, et al. A disease locus for familial hypertrophic cardiomyopathy maps to chromosome 1q3. Nat Genet 1993; 3:333-7.
8. Thierfelder L, MacRae C, Watkins H, et al. A familial hypertrophic cardiomyopathy locus maps to chromosome 15q2. Proc Natl Acad Sci USA. 1993; 90:6270-4.
9. Carrier L, Hengstenberg C, Beckmann JS, et al. Mapping of a novel gene for familial hypertrophic cardiomyopathy to chromosome 11. Nat Genet 1993; 4:311-3.
10. MacRae CA, Ghaisas N, Kass S, et al. Familial hypertrophic cardiomyopathy with Wolff-Parkinson-White Syndrome maps to a locus on chromosome 7q3. J Clin Invest 1995;96:1216-20.
11. Poetter K, Jiang H, Hassanzadeh S, et al. Mutation in either the essential or regulatory light chains of myosin are associated with a rare myopathy in human heart and skeletal muscle. Nat Genet 1996;13:63-9.
12. Kimura A, Harada H, Park JE, et al. Mutations in the cardiac troponin I gene associated with hypertrophic cardiomyopathy. Nat Genet 1997;16:379-82.
13. Bonne G, Carrier L, Richard P, Hainque B, Schwartz K. Familial hypertrophic cardiomyopathy from mutations to functional defects. Circ Res 1998; 83:580-93.
14. Hofmann PA, Hartzell HC, Moss RL. Alterations in Ca^{2+} sensitive tension due to partial extraction of C-protein from rat skinned cardiac myocytes and rabbit skeletal muscle fibers. J Gen Physiol 1991;97:1141-63.
15. Carrier L, Bonne G, Bährend E, et al. Organization and sequence of human cardiac myosin binding protein C gene (MYBPC3) and identification of mutations predicted to produce truncated proteins in familial hypertrophic cardiomyopathy. Circ Res 1997;80:427-34.
16. Gautel M, Zuffardi O, Freiburg A, Labeit S. Phosphorylation switches specific for the cardiac isoform of myosin binding protein C: a modulator of cardiac contraction? EMBO J 1995;14:1952-60.
17. Fougerousse F, Delezoide AL, Fiszman MY, Schwartz K, Beckmann JS, Carrier L. Cardiac myosin binding protein C gene is specifically expressed in heart during murine and human development. Circ Res 1998;82:130-3.
18. Gautel M, Fürst DO, Cocco A, Schiaffino S. Isoform transitions of the myosin-binding protein C family in developing human and mouse muscles. Lack of isoform transcomplementation in cardiac muscle. Circ Res 1998;82:124-9.
19. Mesnard L, Logeart D, Taviaux S, Diriong S, Mercadier JJ, Samson F. Human cardiac troponin T: cloning and expression of new isoforms in the normal and failing heart. Circ Res 1995;76:687-92.
20. Townsend P, Barton P, Yacoub M, Farza H. Molecular cloning of human cardiac troponin T isoforms: expression in developing and failing heart. J Mol Cell Cardiol 1995;27:2223-36.
21. Forissier JF, Carrier L, Farza H, et al. Codon 102 of the cardiac troponin T gene is a putative hot spot for mutations in familial hypertrophic cardiomyopathy. Circulation 1996;94:3069-73.
22. Farza H, Townsend PJ, Cariier L, et al. Genomic organisation, alternative splicing and polymorphisms of the human cardiac trophin T gene. J Mol Cell Cardiol 1998; 30:1247-53.
23. Jones W, Grupp I, Doetschman T, et al. Ablation of the murine alpha myosin heavy chain gene leads to dosage effects and functional deficits in the heart. J Clin Invest 1996;98:
24. Nishi H, Kimura A, Harada H, et al. A myosin missense mutation, not a null allele, causes familial hypertrophic cardiomyopathy. Circulation 1995;91:2911-5.
25. Watkins H, Seidman CE, Seidman JG, Feng HS, Sweeney HL. Expression and functional assessment of a truncated cardiac troponin T that causes hypertrophic cardiomyopathy. J Clin Invest 1996;98:2456-61.
26. Rottbauer W, Gautel M, Zehelein J, et al. Novel splice donor site mutation in the cardiac myosin-binding protein-C gene in familial hypertrophic cardiomyopathy. Characterization of cardiac transcript and protein. J

Clin Invest 1997;100:475-82.

27. Spirito P, Seidman CE, Mckenna WJ, Maron BJ. The management of hypertrophic cardiomyopathy. N Engl J Med 1997;336:775-85.

28. Moolman JC, Corfield VA, Posen B, et al. Sudden death due to troponin T mutations. J Am Coll Cardiol 1997;29:549-5.

29. Nakajima-Taniguchi C, Matsui H, Fujio Y, Nagata S, Kishimoto T, Yamauchi-Takihara K. Novel missense mutation in cardiac troponin T gene found in japanese patient with hypertrophic cardiomyopathy. J Mol Cell Cardiol 1997;29:839-43.

30. Bonne G, Carrier L, Bercovici J, et al. Cardiac myosin binding protein-C gene splice acceptor site mutation is associated with familial hypertrophic cardiomyopathy. Nat Genet 1995;11:438-40.

31. Watkins H, Conner D, Thierfelder L, et al. Mutations in the cardiac myosin binding protein-C gene on chromosome 11 cause familial hypertrophic cardiomyopathy. Nat Genet 1995;11:434-7.

32. Niimura H, Bachinski LL, Sangwatanaroj S, et al. Mutations in the gene for cardiac myosin-binding protein C and late-onset familial hypertrophic cardiomyopathy. N Engl J Med 1998;338:1248-57.

33. Charron P, Dubourg O, Desnos M, et al. Clinical features and prognostic implications of familial hypertrophic cardiomyopathy related to cardiac myosin binding protein C gene. Circulation 1998; 97:2230-6.

34. Marian AJ, Yu Q-T, Workman R, Greve G, Roberts R. Angiotensin-converting enzyme polymorphism in hypertrophic cardiomyopathy and sudden death. Lancet 1993;342:1085-6.

35. Yonega K, Okamoto H, Machida M, et al. Angiotensin-converting enzyme gene polymorphism in japanese patients with hyeprtrophic cardiomyopathy. Am Heart J 1995;130:1089-93.

36. Tesson F, Dufour C, Moolman JC, et al. The influence of the angiotensin I converting enzyme genotype in familial hypertrophic cardiomyopathy varies with the disease gene mutation. J Mol Cell Cardiol 1997;29:831-8.

37. Sakamoto A, Ono K, Abe M, et al. Both hypertrophic and dilated cardiomyopthies are caused by mutation in the same gene, d-sarcoglycan, in hamster: an animal model of disrupted dystrophin-associated glycoprotein complex. Proc Natl Acad Sci U S A 1997;94:13873-8.

38. Olson TM, Michels VV, Thibodeau SN, Tai YS, Keating MT. Actin mutations in dilated cardiomyopathy, a heritable form of heart failure. Science 1998;280:750-2.

INDEX